Topical Glucocorticoids with Increased Benefit/Risk Ratio

Current Problems in Dermatology

Vol. 21

Series Editor   *G. Burg,* Zurich

KARGER

Basel · Freiburg · Paris · London · New York ·
New Delhi · Bangkok · Singapore · Tokyo · Sydney

Topical Glucocorticoids with Increased Benefit/Risk Ratio

Volume Editors *H.C. Korting,* Munich
H.I. Maibach, San Francisco, Calif.

58 figures, 10 color plates, 47 tables, 1993

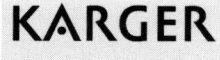

Basel · Freiburg · Paris · London · New York ·
New Delhi · Bangkok · Singapore · Tokyo · Sydney

....
Current Problems in Dermatology

Library of Congress Cataloging-in-Publication Data
Topical glucocorticoids with increased benefit/risk ratio
volume editors, H.C. Korting, H.I. Maibach.
(Current problems in dermatology; vol. 21)
Includes bibliographical references and index.   (alk. paper)
1. Glucocorticoids – Therapeutic use.   2. Transdermal medication.   3. Dermatopharmacology.
I. Korting, Hans Christian.   II. Maibach, Howard I.   III. Series.
[DNLM: 1. Glucocorticoids, Topical.   2. Odds Ratio
W1 CU804L v.21 1993 / QV 60 T673 1992]
RM292.3. T67   1993
615'.364–dc20
ISBN 3–8055–5712–4

Contents

Applied Pharmacologic Considerations

Clinical Considerations

Future Prospects

Preface

The introduction of a topical glucocorticoid, i.e., hydrocortisone, into the treatment of inflammatory skin disease by Sulzberger and Witten in 1952 provided a major pharmacologic breakthrough. In fact, we distinguish two eras of dermatologic treatment, i.e., before and after 'cortisone'. However, it was clear early that hydrocortisone and hydrocortisone acetate alone would not suffice as adequate treatment for all types of inflammatory skin disease. Fortunately, other glucocorticoids such as fluorinated congeners offered additional potency. Yet as early as in 1964, Epstein et al. described 'atrophic striae' due to the application of triamcinolone acetonide; many other local adverse effects have subsequently been documented. Even more potent glucocorticoids, e.g., clobetasol propionate, gave us still more efficacy. However, this was linked to more and more severe adverse effects both of the local and the systemic type.

For decades topical glucocorticoids represent the class of topical dermatics most often used, and, in fact, it is not mainly hydrocortisone that is prescribed in daily practice but the more potent congeners. Thus it does not come as a surprise that today the typical adverse effects due to topical glucocorticoids are well known to patients. In fact, some are so scared that the term 'corticophobia' has been proposed. An exaggerated fear of topical glucocorticoids in general, however, can have severe consequences if, for example, severe atopic eczema which can lead to growth retardation is not adequately treated in childhood.

In recent years it has been a challenge both to the chemists and the dermatologists to develop glucocorticoids which are potent but to at least a lesser extent linked to systemic and/or local unwanted effects.

Several years ago, prednicarbate became available, and since the early days of its clinical application, some dermatologists shared the belief that this compound might be different. Chemically, it can be considered a nonhalogenated double-ester type glucocorticoid. More recently, further substances of this type have been synthesized and offered to the clinician. These compounds are not derived from prednisolone but from hydrocortisone. Reflecting their chemical structures they have been named hydrocortisone aceponate and hydrocortisone buteprate. Nevertheless, up to the present, some students of the field still believe that topical glucocorticoids only differ in potency.

A comprehensive monograph on the broad field of 'topical corticosteroids' in general was published recently [Maibach HI, Surber C (eds): Topical Corticosteroids. Basel, Karger, 1992]; the present volume focuses on its subject in a more limited sense. Thus it can be concise; this makes the editors hope that it will be read by many dermatologists – not only those in research but also those in clinical practice. This might spread information on a new approach which may offer the possibility of decreased adverse effects.

Munich/San Francisco, Calif.

Hans C. Korting, MD
Howard I. Maibach, MD

Korting HC, Maibach HI (eds): Topical Glucocorticoids with Increased Benefit/Risk Ratio.
Curr Probl Dermatol. Basel, Karger, 1993, vol 21, pp 1–10

....

Do We Need New and Different Glucocorticoids?

A Re-Appraisal of the Various Congeners and Potential Alternatives

Eric W. Smith

School of Pharmaceutical Sciences, Rhodes University, Grahamstown, South Africa

Historical Aspects

The introduction of hydrocortisone into topical therapy in 1952 initiated a revolution in the treatment of dermatological (especially eczematous) conditions that had been only poorly managed up to that time. The success observed with Kendall's compound F [1] followed several investigations using cortisone and its acetate ester [2, 3] which demonstrated little topical efficacy. It is interesting to note that even in these early years clinicians were concerned about the possible adverse effects following systemic absorption of glucocorticoids [4]. The years between 1952 and 1954 witnessed increasing use of hydrocortisone and its acetate ester in general clinical practice [5, 6] and also in paediatric practice [7]. However, it was soon noted that hydrocortisone was relatively ineffective in the treatment of psoriasis, contact dermatitis and other inflammatory conditions (which we now understand to be generated by different inflammatory mechanisms).

In an attempt to increase the potency of hydrocortisone (and, hopefully, its spectrum of clinical usefulness), the 9α-fluoro derivative (fluorohydrocortisone) was introduced in 1955 [8] and the systemic side effects of this halogenated form were soon documented [9]. Alternatively, introduction of a double bond in the A ring of the molecule also improved potency as demonstrated by prednisolone [10]. A combination of fluorination, A ring dehydrogenation and esterification of the D ring in triamcinolone acetonide produced a structure that was very potent in comparison to the original hydrocortisone. The introduction of this drug into

Table 1. Chronological introduction of topical corticosteroids into clinical practice

Year	Steroid
1950–52	Cortisone, cortisone acetate
1952	Hydrocortisone (Kendall's compound F)
1955	Fluorohydrocortisone, prednisone
1958	Triamcinolone acetonide
1959	Fluorometholone
1960–61	*Occlusive application techniques*
1961	Fluocinolone acetonide, fluorandrenolone
1962	Dexamethasone
1963	**Betamethasone dipropionate**
1966	Flumethasone pivalate
1969	**Clobetasol propionate**
1970	**Desoximetasone,** hydrocortisone butyrate
1971	Fluocinonide
1972	Halcinonide, betamethasone benzoate
1976	Amcinonide, desonide, **diflorasone diacetate**
1978	Hydrocortisone valerate, budesonide
1982	Alcomethasone dipropionate
1985	Prednicarbate
1988	Mometasone furoate

Superpotent corticoids are indicated in bold.

clinical practice in 1958 [11] probably marked the start of the era of superpotent topical corticosteroids, the numbers of which were to swell markedly in the next 2 decades. Additional methylation of the B ring also improved clinical efficacy as exemplified by fluorometholone which was introduced in 1959 [12]. To increase the efficacy of these agents even further, application sites were occluded with water-impervious material. Several reports appeared in the literature during the next few years describing occlusive techniques that prevented moisture evaporation [13] or supplied water to hydrate the stratum corneum [14], both methods enhancing steroid permeation.

During the period 1960–1980 a number of glucocorticoid analogues (table 1) were synthesized and evaluated for topical anti-inflammatory activity. The initial synthetic thrust was to produce halogenated, dehydrogenated and esterified molecules that were intrinsically of high lipophilicity and potency, clobetasol propionate being representative of the more potent of these agents. The severe adverse reactions generated by these potent compounds [15, 16] have changed the research impetus in recent years to synthesizing molecules that have anti-inflammatory activity without the unwanted systemic and local side-effects. Agents such as budesonide or prednicarbate are reported to demonstrate some success in this regard by maintaining glucocorticoid potency without the need for B ring halogenation.

Glucocorticoid Chemistry

All steroids exhibiting glucocorticoid (and mineralocorticoid) activity are derived from the 21-carbon pregnane series parent molecule (fig. 1) and all have a double bond at position 4 (pregn-4-ene). The potency of these molecules is dependent on the nature and site of substitution on this steroid skeleton. Substituents may increase potency by increasing the lipophilic properties of the molecule, thereby making them more permeable to biological membranes, by increasing the corticoid-receptor binding affinity or by delaying metabolism of the molecule once absorbed.

Hydrocortisone has 2 ketone (C-3, C-20) and 3 hydroxy (C-11, C-17, C-21) groups and demonstrates relatively low potency and a short duration of action. Introduction of an additional double bond at C-1 (e.g. prednisolone) decreases mineralocorticoid activity (oedema and hypertension) and enhances glucocorticoid effects. Additional glucocorticoid specificity is achieved by substitution at the C-16 position; triamcinolone and betamethasone, for example, have little mineralocorticoid activity.

Lipophilicity and duration of action is greatly increased by halogenation (usually fluorination) of the B ring at the C-9 position (triamcinolone), at the C-6 position (fluprednisolone) or both the C-6 and C-9 positions (diflucortolone). The lipophilicity and metabolic resistance of the glucocorticoids may also be increased by the addition of ester or acetal groups to the D ring. The most common groups employed for this purpose are acetate, propionate, butyrate, valerate and pivalate esters and the acetonide acetal group (fig. 2). Betamethasone 17-valerate, clobetasol 17-propionate and fluocinolone acetonide are typical examples of these chemical modifications. Substitution in this manner usually has a marked effect on potency: betamethasone is approximately 10 times more potent than hydrocortisone, while the valerate derivative of betamethasone is approximately 300 times more potent than hydrocortisone.

Based on these chemical modifications and the duration of action of the agents, the topical corticosteroids have been classified in terms of their potency (table 2). Clinicians may make reference to this classification when considering suitable drugs to treat a particular dermatological condition. It is interesting to note that some classifications list the same drug in different potency classifications depending on the delivery vehicle used. A particular drug may elicit a

PREGN - 4 - ENE

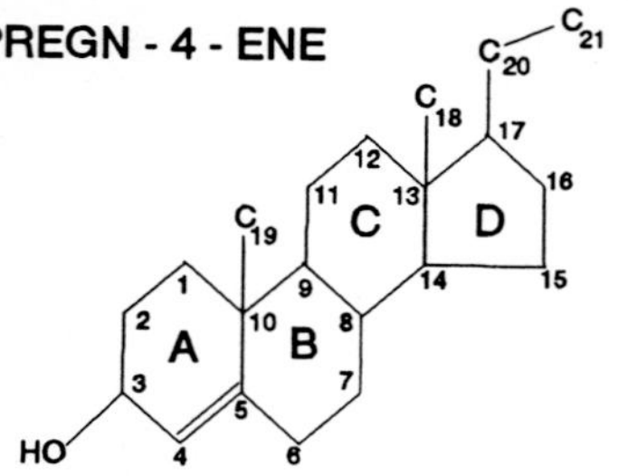

HYDROCORTISONE
(CORTISOL)

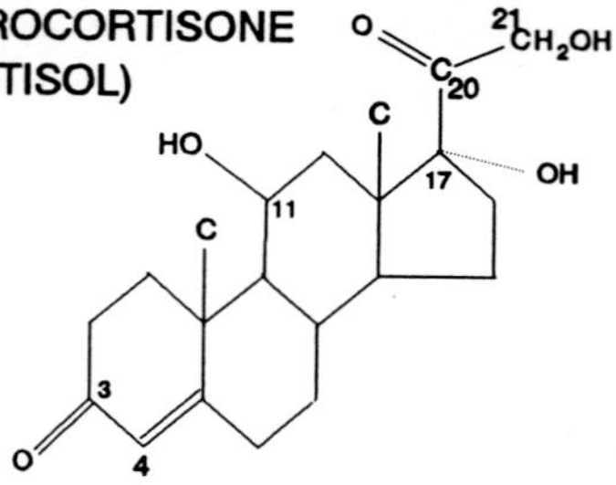

PREDNISOLONE
↑ mineralocorticoid
↑ glucocorticoid

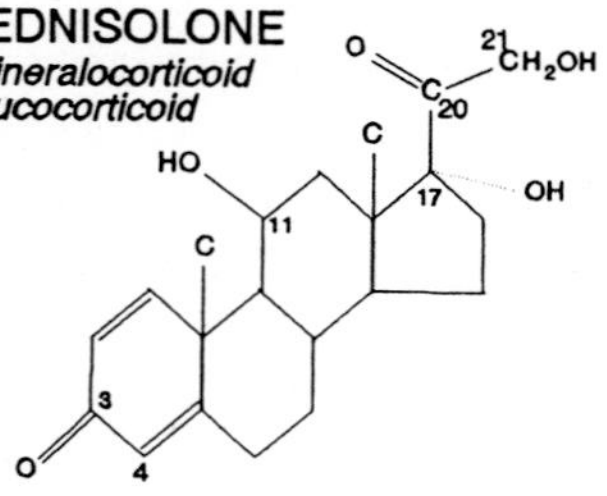

TRIAMCINOLONE
↑ glucocorticoid

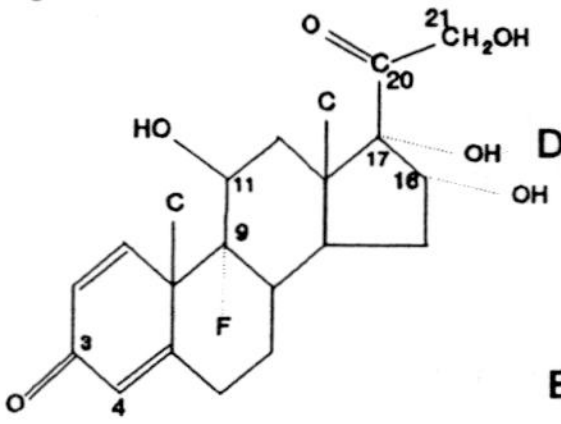

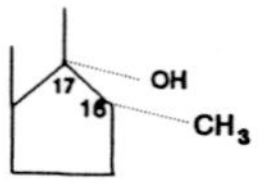

Dexamethasone

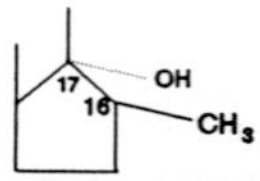

Betamethasone

FLUPREDNISOLONE

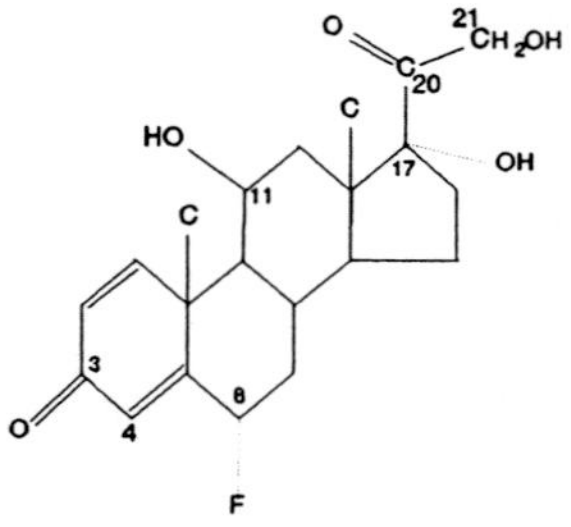

DIFLUCORTOLONE

↑ glucocorticoid

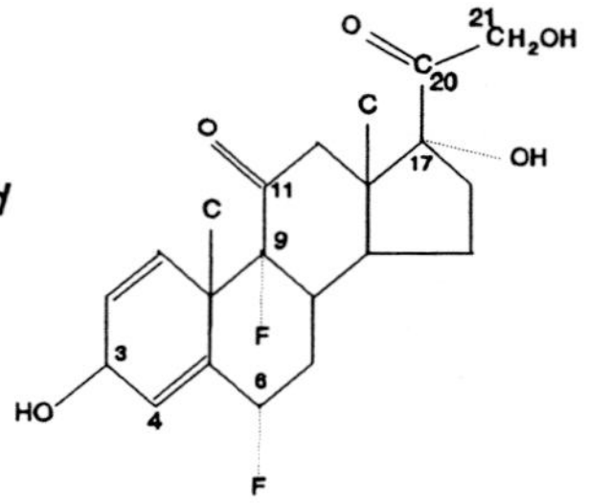

BETAMETHASONE
17- VALERATE

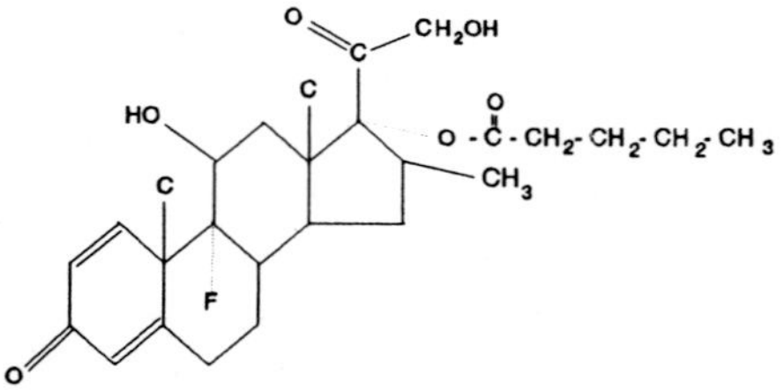

CLOBETASOL
PROPIONATE

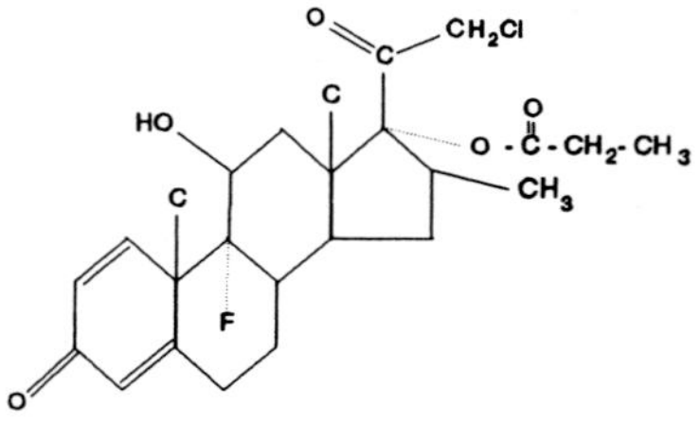

1

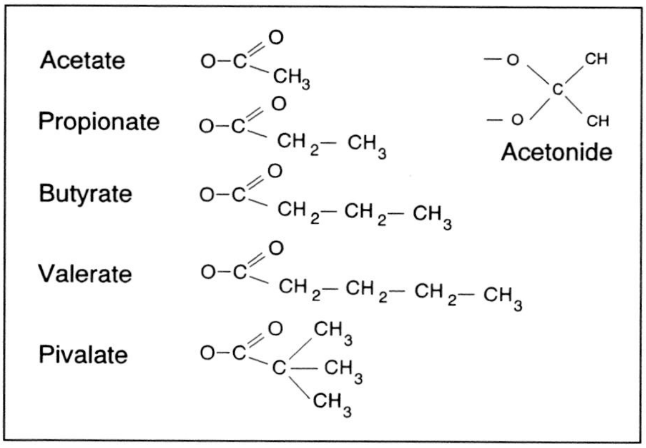

Fig. 2. Ester and acetal groups commonly used for increasing lipophilicity and activity of topical corticosteroids.

Table 2. Potency classification of common topical corticosteroids

Very potent	*Moderately potent*
Clobetasol propionate 0.05%	Clobetasone butyrate 0.05%
Fluocinolone acetonide 0.2%	Fluocinolone acetonide 0.01%
Beclomethasone dipropionate 0.5%	Flucortolone
Diflucortolone valerate 0.3%	Methylprednisolone acetate
Halcinonide 0.1%	
	Weak
Potent	Hydrocortisone
Beclomethasone dipropionate 0.025%	Hydrocortisone acetate
Betamethasone 17-valerate	Methylprednisolone
Desonide 0.05%	
Diflucortolone valerate 0.1%	
Fluclorolone acetonide 0.025%	
Fluocinolone acetonide 0.025%	
Fluocinonide 0.05%	
Flumethasone pivalate 0.02%	
Fluprednylidine acetate 0.1%	
Halcinonide 0.1%	
Hydrocortisone butyrate 0.1%	
Triamcinolone acetonide	

Fig. 1. Molecular modifications of pregnene that progressively increase glucocorticoid potency.

greater potency when delivered, for example, in an ointment vehicle compared to a cream base, or in alcoholic solution compared to a lotion formulation. Cognisance of the effects of the vehicle in delivering the drug are as important for the dermatologist as is the choice of which drug to use. Formulation pharmacists also argue about the merits of diluting a potent product [17] (thereby changing the stability and delivery environment for the drug that has been painstakingly researched and optimized) when there are commercial products of lower potency that could be prescribed instead that would probably generate an identical therapeutic effect. The anatomical site to which the drug is to be applied is also important. It has long been documented [18] that some regions of the body allow greater transfer of corticosteroids than do others; the use of high-potency drugs on skin regions of high permeability is unwarranted.

Adverse Reactions of Topical Glucocorticoids

Topical glucocorticoids are multipotent agonists that influence a multitude of interconnected biochemical pathways in a complex manner, the full understanding of which is still in its infancy. The synthetic problem that has faced the pharmaceutical chemist in the past 4 decades is the attempted separation of these effects by molecular modification. The lack of success in this regard currently appears to be due to the non-specificity of the glucocorticoid receptor. The conformation (and therefore the intracellular activity) of the activated steroid-receptor complex appears to be independent of the specific glucocorticoid molecule binding with the receptor [19]. This would suggest that corticoid potency is more related to metabolic resistance and increased lipophilicity rather than receptor dynamics.

The main mode of topical anti-inflammatory activity is currently believed to be through inhibition of phospholipase A_2, an enzyme responsible for the formation of prostaglandins, leukotrienes and other pro-inflammatory hydroxy fatty acids from arachidonic acid (fig. 3). Binding of the glucocorticoid to its receptor in the cytosol is followed by translocation of the drug-receptor complex to the nuclear DNA where normal protein transcription via mRNA stimulates synthesis of an antiphospholipase A_2 protein, lipocortin, within the ribosomes. The catalytic effects of phospholipase A_2 in the production of the inflammatory mediators is almost completely blocked by lipocortin in the presence of exogenous corticosteroids. There are undoubtedly other mediator pathways that are also affected by the steroid presence in the epidermal and dermal cells. The migration and activity of phagocytes and other inflammatory mediators is suppressed (inflammatory dermatoses), production of lymphocytes, monocytes and polymorphonuclear granulocytes decreases and autolysis via lysosomes is depressed. Fibrin and colla-

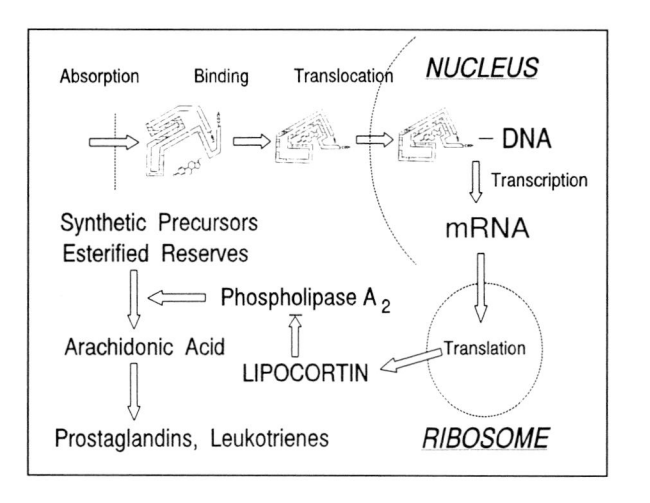

Fig. 3. Schematic mechanism of action of glucocorticoids in the cytosol.

gen deposition is inhibited, cell mitosis and maturation is delayed (proliferative dermatoses) and capillary dilation and permeability are increased.

In many cases the improved therapeutic value of these potent agents has been overshadowed by the serious side-effects experienced by patients, these reactions ranging in severity from skin thinning to full hypothalamic-pituitary axis suppression (table 3). The severity of these adverse reactions correlates with the potency of the corticoid employed, the duration of therapy and the use of occlusion or occlusive delivery vehicles. Thinning (usually reversible) of the epidermis and dermis is almost universal when potent glucocorticoids are used, especially in children or where occlusive application regimens have been employed, and is usually discernable days after therapy is initiated [20]. Subcutaneous blood vessels may become visible through the thinned skin (telangiectasia) which is more susceptible to physical trauma and fissure formation. Irreversible skin striae often develop in the limb flexures or under occluded application of potent corticoids. Purpuric patches may also develop due to the loss of supportive tissue surrounding the vasculature. Many of these effects are thought to be due to reduced dermal collagen and an inhibition of fibroblast activity which reduces formation of new collagen.

The inflammatory response following microbial infection of the skin may be suppressed by corticosteroids, allowing the pathogen greater freedom to proliferate in the absence of the body's defence mechanism. Impairment of the body's ability to sequestrate the pathogen may result in rapid spread of the infection to other body sites. Many dermatological, especially psoriatic, conditions may flare

Table 3. Adverse side effects of topical glucocorticoid therapy

Peripheral adverse reactions	*Systemic adverse reactions*
Skin atrophy	Suppression of hypothalamic-pituitary-
Thinning	adrenal axis
Telangiectasia	Depressed ACTH production
Fissures and tearing	Impaired stress response
Striae (flexures)	Iatrogenic Cushing's syndrome
Blood vessel dilation	Hyperglycaemia
Purpura	(Increased production,
Photosensitization	decreased utilization)
Masked microbial infections	Impaired protein catabolism
Rebound flare (psoriasis)	(Muscle atrophy)
Steroid acne	Lipid store relocation
Ophthalmic pathologies	(Hyperlipidaemia)
	Renal impairment
	(Oedema, hypertension)

up in a rebound fashion on cessation of treatment, this situation often being treated with more potent agents or more drastic application regimens. Acne may be induced or exacerbated by corticosteroid application as may diverse ophthalmic pathologies following ocular absorption.

Systemic side-effects are generally of a more serious nature. Suppression of the hypothalamic-pituitary-adrenal axis (manifesting as oedema, cushingoid features, hyperglycaemia and glycosuria) is a homeostatic negative feedback response to the high systemic glucocorticoid concentrations following extensive transdermal absorption [15]. Absorption of the drug in sufficient amounts to induce this effect can easily be achieved in infants or where potent corticosteroids have been chronically applied in large doses (often with occlusion) to inflamed skin which is inherently more permeable than healthy tissue. A dose of 14 g/week of clobetasol propionate or 49 g/week of betamethasone dipropionate is sufficient to suppress plasma cortisol levels. Similarly, iatrogenic Cushing's syndrome [21], involving several diverse organ systems, may result from prolonged exposure to potent glucocorticoids and may cause growth suppression in children [22]. Metabolic side effects following topical corticosteroid application are numerous and affect diverse tissue systems. Increased glucose production and decreased glucose utilization induce hyperglycaemia and may lead to diabetes mellitus. Adverse protein catabolism results in muscle and skin atrophy and may lead to osteoporosis. Lipid stores are relocated from the limbs to the face, neck and trunk, often associated with increased blood titres of circulating triglycerides.

Conclusions

Dermatology has undergone a major revolution with the introduction of topical corticosteroid therapy. Modification of the basic pregnane steroid structure by A ring dehydrogenation, B ring halogenation and esterification or acetal addition to the D ring have greatly increased the lipophilicity and clinical potency of the glucocorticoid molecules. Newer and more potent drugs have improved the spectrum of topical diseases that may be treated by the clinician. However, there has been much adverse reaction, both public and professional, to the unwanted side-effects of the more potent formulations in general use and many patients have been reluctant to use these preparations. More conservative usage of these drugs in recent years has helped restore confidence in topical corticosteroid therapy.

In answer to the question whether we need new and different glucocorticoids, we can now answer emphatically that we do not need more potent drugs; we need drugs that can more effectively separate wanted anti-inflammatory effects from unwanted side-effects. Binding of the corticoid to the peripheral receptor elicits a multitude of different responses which have, as yet, been inadequately separable by chemical modification. Undoubtedly as specialist knowledge in this field increases this goal appears more achievable in the future. Alternatively, we should perhaps focus our attention on other drug entities that act at other points in the inflammatory mediator cascade and which present less potential for adverse side-effects. In the interim, a more judicious use of the different potency classes of corticoid, different delivery vehicles for the same corticoid and the optimization of alternating dosage regimens may prevent many of the more serious untoward effects of this class of drugs.

Acknowledgements

The financial assistance from Rhodes University Council, the Foundation for Research Development and Cassella-Riedel Pharma GmbH is acknowledged with gratitude.

References

1   Sulzberger MB, Witten VH: Effect of topically applied compound F in selected dermatoses. J Invest Dermatol 1952;19:101–102.
2   Newman BA, Feldman FF: Effects of topical cortisone on chronic discoid lupus erythematosus and necrobiosis lipoidica diabeticorum. J Invest Dermatol 1951;17:3–6.
3   Goldman L, Thompson RG, Trice ER: Cortisone acetate in skin disease: Local effect in skin from topical applications and local injection. Arch Dermatol Syph 1951;19:101–102.
4   Smith CC: Eosinophilic response after inunction of hydrocortisone ointment: Experiments demonstrating lack of significant absorption and of systemic effects. Arch Dermatol Syph 1953;68:50–53.

5   Grupper C: Local applications of hydrocortisone in dermatology. Bull Soc Franc Dermatol Syph 1953;60:474–478.
6   Robinson HM, Robinson RCV: Treatment of dermatoses with local application of hydrocortisone acetate. JAMA 1954;115:1213–1216.
7   McCorriston LR: Hydrocortisone (compound F) acetate ointment in eczema of infants and children. Can Med Assoc J 1954;70:59–62.
8   Witten VH, Sulzberger MB, Zimmerman EH, Shapiro AJ: Therapeutic assay of topically applied 9αfluorohydrocortisone acetate in selected dermatoses. J Invest Dermatol 1955;24:1–4.
9   Fitzpatrick TB, Griswold HC, Hicks JH: Sodium retention and edema from percutaneous absorption of fludrocortisone acetate. JAMA 1955;158:1149–1152.
10   Frank L, Stritzler C: Prednisolone topically and systemically: Clinical evaluation in selective dermatoses (preliminary report). Arch Dermatol 1955;72:547–549.
11   Robinson RCV: Treatment of dermatoses with local application of triamcinolone acetonide, a new synthetic corticoid: Preliminary report. Bull School Med Univ Md 1958;43:54–57.
12   Cahn MM, Levy EJ: A comparison of topical corticosteroids: Triamcinolone acetonide, prednisolone, fluorometholone and hydrocortisone. Antibiot Med 1959;6:734.
13   Sulzberger MB, Witten VH: Thin pliable plastic films in topical dermatologic therapy. Arch Dermatol 1961;84:1027–1028.
14   Tye MJ, Schiff BL: Treatment of psoriatic lesions with topical fluocinolone acetonide moist dressings. J Invest Dermatol 1962;38:321–322.
15   Stoughton RCD, August PJ: Cushing's syndrome and pituitary-adrenal suppression due to clobetasol propionate. Br Med J 1975;2:419–421.
16   Novak E, Schlagei CA, Sechman CE, Chen TT: Diflorasone diacetate: Adrenal suppression and systemic tolerance study in normal human volunteers. Curr Ther Res 1980;26:562–569.
17   Clement M, du Vivier A: Concern about the current clinical practice of diluting topical glucocorticosteroid preparations. Clin Exp Dermatol 1984;9:323–324.
18   Feldmann RJ, Maibach HI: Regional variation in percutaneous penetration of ^{14}C cortisol in man. J Invest Dermatol 1967;48:181–183.
19   Zeelen FJ: Medicinal chemistry of steroids: Recent developments. Adv Drug Res 1992;22:149–189.
20   Lubach D, Grüter H, Behl M, Nagel C: Investigations on the development and regression of corticosteroid-induced thinning of the skin in various parts of the human body during and after topical application of amcinonide. Dermatologica 1989;178:93–97.
21   May P, Stein ES, Ryter RJ, Hirsh FS, Michel B, Levy RP: Cushing's syndrome from percutaneous absorption of triamcinolone cream. Arch Intern Med 1976;136:612–613.
22   Vermeer BJ, Heremans GFP: A case of growth retardation and Cushing's syndrome due to excessive application of betamethasone-17-valerate ointment. Dermatologica 1974;149:299–304.

Eric W. Smith, PhD, School of Pharmaceutical Sciences, Rhodes University,
PO Box 94, Grahamstown 6140 (South Africa)

Korting HC, Maibach HI (eds): Topical Glucocorticoids with Increased Benefit/Risk Ratio.
Curr Probl Dermatol. Basel, Karger, 1993, vol 21, pp 11–19

Design of Novel Soft Corticosteroids

Nicholas Bodor

Center for Drug Discovery, University of Florida, Gainesville, Fla., USA

It is well known that glucocorticoid therapy includes a variety of useful applications related to the multiple activity of this class of compounds. These include anti-inflammatory, antiallergic, immunosuppressor or antitumor activities, and the respective uses cover rheumatoid arthritis, systemic lupus, cancer in certain leukemias, immunosuppressing effects in grafts and, probably most importantly, the various topical applications, including dermatitis and other disorders of the skin, colon (for the treatment of colitis) and asthma by inhalation. Due to the ubiquitous nature of the glucocorticoid receptors and the intrinsic multiple activity of glucocorticoids, associated with most useful applications are a number of unwanted side effects. Most of these are receptor-mediated, and are typical corticosteroid effects, such as suppression of the pituitary-adrenal axis. Other side effects, including growth inhibition in children or skin thinning during topical application, in addition to systemic side effects, could present serious problems. There are also some specific side effects not directly related to receptor binding properties which are, however, connected to the specific structure of the glucocorticoids, such as reactions with various macromolecules, which were implicated in such side effects such as cataract formation.

For many years, the main strategies in designing improved corticosteroids concentrated on molecular manipulation of the basic steroidal structure in order to enhance one or the other specific activity. Indeed, by modifying various sites at the basic corticosteroid molecule, ultrapotent corticosteroids were developed with improved glucocorticoid activity. However, the most important side effects have persisted and in most cases actually have increased parallel with the increase in the desired activities. It appeared, then, that new types of approaches are needed to be able to separate the desired activity and the multiple toxicity properties of glucocorticoids.

During the past decade or so, new approaches in improving the therapeutic index of drugs have been developed, based on involving drug metabolism considerations at an early stage of drug design. These are combined under the generic name of *retrometabolic drug design methods* which include [1] two major classes: one is the metabolic activation by design of inactive chemical delivery forms, called *'chemical delivery systems'* and the other is the opposite of this, that is, controlled metabolic deactivation of specifically designed active species, called *'soft drugs'*. These latter, the soft-drug concepts, were extensively used in designing new classes of corticosteroids [2], based on the *'inactive metabolite approach'*. According to the retrometabolic design by soft drugs, the objective is to design safe and better drugs by controlled and directed drug metabolism. Thus, soft drugs are new chemical compounds characterized by a predictable and controllable in vivo deactivation (metabolism to nontoxic inactive moieties) after they achieve their therapeutic role.

Design and Evaluation of Some Soft Corticosteroids

The first major implication of these concepts is the deliberate simplification of the metabolism of the drugs, that is, instead of the usual multiple metabolic activation-deactivation, the objective of drug design by soft drugs is a facile, preferable one-step complete deactivation of the drug after it leaves the site of action, which is generally the site where it is applied. Among the various specific design methods, the inactive metabolite approach was most successful in designing soft corticosteroids [2]. In this case, the design starts from a known inactive metabolite of a drug which is used as a lead compound. The inactive metabolite then is modified strategically in order to produce an isosteric and/or isoelectronic analogue of the active lead compound, in this way assuming the activity. The most important second aspect of the design is, however, that a predictable and rate-controlled metabolism will yield the very starting inactive metabolite. In this case, one can predict and control the activity-toxicity away from the site of action. Of course, the transport and binding properties of the new soft drugs, as well as the rate of metabolism, will determine the ultimate success, and these are the subject of the specific molecular manipulation attempts.

We have previously reported an application of the inactive metabolite approach to the glucocorticoids, where among the various active and inactive metabolites of the basic glucocorticoid, hydrocortisone (structure *1*, fig. 1), the inactive metabolite cortienic acid (structure *2*, fig. 1) was selected as the lead compound. Accordingly, the cortienic acid and its various ring-substituted analogues were converted by modification of the acidic and other functions to provide a set of isosteric/isoelectronic molecules, structurally close to some of the most potent

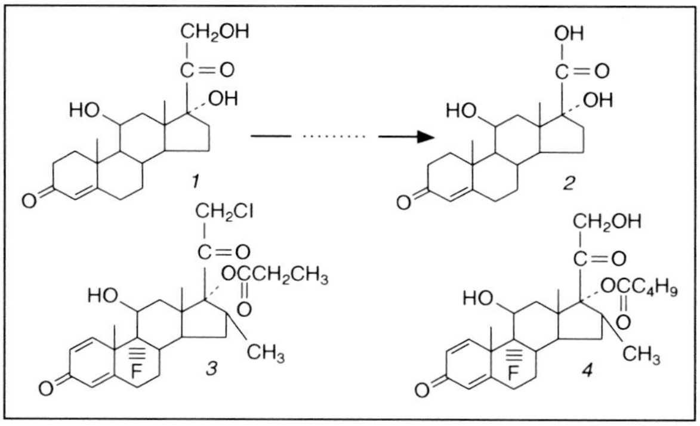

Fig. 1. Design principles of the soft corticosteroids. The lead compound is the inactive cortienic acid (*2*) metabolite of hydrocortisone (*1*). Isosteric/isoelectronic modifications of 2, based on structural features of potent glucocorticoids, like clobetasol propionate (*3*) and betamethasone valerate (*4*), result in the soft analogs listed in table 1.

glucocorticoids, such as clobetasol propionate (structure *3*, fig. 1), betamethasone valerate (structure *4*, fig. 1), and others.

The specific modifications which led to the best soft compounds include 17α-carbonate and 17α-ether derivatives of the cortienic acid esters, containing an α-heteroatom, such as the chloro- and fluoromethyl derivatives. The advantage of the 17α-carbonates over 17α-carboxylesters is in the relative stability of the carbonate function as opposed to the simple esters, thus preventing formation of the mixed anhydrides [2] and subsequent reaction with nucleophiles in the cell components. It is also important to note that the new class of compounds, lacking the 20 ketones, which was implicated in the formation of cataracts (Hines rearrangement [2] and references cited), is also avoided. The general class of the cortienic-acid-based soft steroids is depicted as structure *5* in figure 2, and the expected and predicted simple deactivation indicates the return to the lead cortienic acid derivatives *6* and *7* (fig. 2).

As shown before [2], specific studies on the separation of anti-inflammatory activity of these new soft steroids compared to the side effects as reflected by the thymolytic activity indicate a dramatic increase in the therapeutic index. Subcutaneous implant of cotton pellets containing various modified soft analogues proved to be as or more effective than hydrocortisone 17α-butyrate or betamethasone valerate in inhibiting granulation, while having virtually no effect on the thymus weight.

The most recent studies concentrated on determining the intrinsic activity of these new soft steroids by establishing their glucocorticoid receptor binding affin-

Design of Novel Soft Corticosteroids

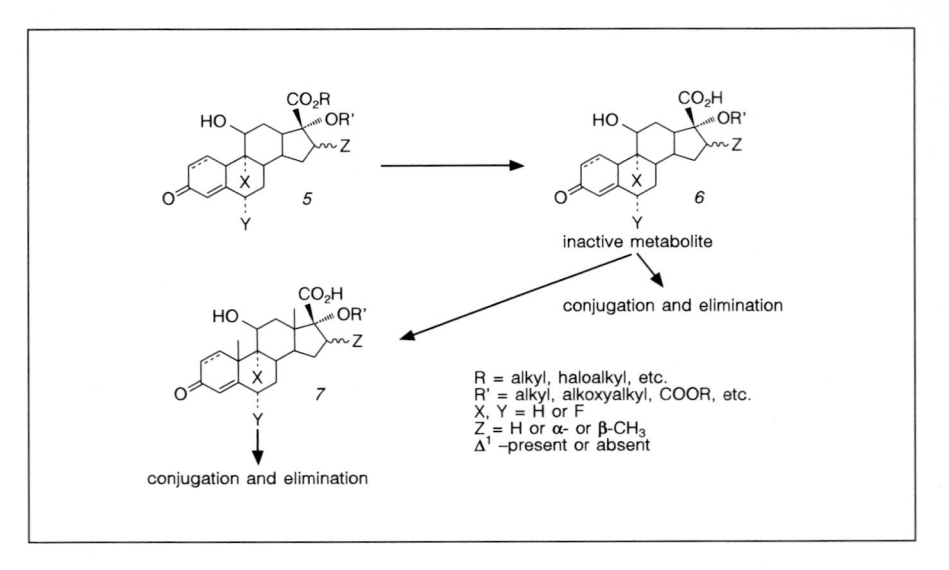

Fig. 2. Based on the soft-drug principles, the designed soft steroids represented by the general structure 5 undergo one step hydrolytic deactivation to the inactive cortienic acid derivatives 6 and 7.

ity, using rat lung type II cytosol receptors [3]. It was hoped that these studies would help in defining the most important structural features in this new class of compounds. The method used dexamethasone as the standard comparison, and the relative binding affinity (RBA) of this reference compound was assigned 100. The specific method used could very well reproduce the RBA of known 'hard' corticosteroids, such as hydrocortisone 17α-butyrate (RBA = 55) or betamethasone 17α-valerate (RBA = 820).

As a first objective, the various acidic metabolites-lead compounds 6 (fig. 2) were studied. There were 27 different acidic metabolites investigated, which contain substituents like the Δ^1, the 9α- and/or 6α-fluorine, 16α- or β-methyl and various 17α-carbonate functions. It was found that all these acids have an RBA less than 1, that is, they are all virtually inactive, in agreement with the design principles. It was found that the introduction of simple alkyl ester function in the molecule (for example, 5, R = methyl or ethyl; fig. 2) did not lead to active compounds even by introducing a 9α-fluoro function. The introduction of some heteroatoms in the ester side chain, for example, the methyl thiomethyl function (8, R = CH_2SCH_3, 17α-ethyl carbonate of cortienic acid) led to minimal activity (RBA = 3). On the other hand, introducing heteroatoms, like chlorine or oxygen, in the relatively short 17α side chains did not much affect the activity, if the 17β-esters were the simple alkyl ones, but it became evident that heteroatoms, such as chlorine in the ester function, have a dramatic effect.

While the chloromethyl esters of 17α-carbonates now demonstrated significant activity as shown in table 1 (structures *9–11*), it became evident that the chloromethyl esters are much more potent than very close analogues like the chloroethylidine, *12* (methyl chloromethyl) or the straight homologues, the chlorethyl *13* esters. As expected, the 11-ketone derivatives are much less active than the desired 11β-OH ones, as shown by comparing structures *14* and *15*. Based on these, a variety of highly potent compounds were developed, all of which are various 17α-carbonates and the substitutions at the 16,6α–9α and Δ¹ position vary as shown by structures *16–21*.

A number of these compounds shows higher intrinsic activity than betamethasone valerate, and it became evident that the fluoromethyl esters (*22* and *23*, even the nonfluorinated *24* and *25*) are essentially as potent as the corresponding chloromethyl analogues. One of these compounds, structure *26*, where the simple 17α-ethyl carbonate is combined with the 16α-methyl and 6α- and 9α-fluorine functions and Δ¹, shows an RBA = 2,100, which in our hands is *the most potent glucocorticoid* ever looked at. The relative effect of the carbonate function in the 17α position is illustrated by the methyl, ethyl and propyl sequence *27, 28* and *29*, where the increase in the chain length to the propyl results in increased activity. All of these analogues, although nonfluorinated, show significantly higher activity than dexamethasone. These compounds which could be considered derived from the inactive metabolite of prednisolone show higher than an order of magnitude increase in the activity over prednisolone itself. It is no surprise that the free 17α-OH derivatives (*30* and *31*) show only minimal activity. As mentioned before, the position of the chlorine in the ester function clearly affects activity. The chloroethyl analogue *13* is more than 35 times less potent than the corresponding chloromethyl ester, *14*. In order to shed some light on the importance of the various heteroatoms in the molecules and, in particular, the substitution in the 21 position as compared to the heteroatom in the ester part of the soft analogues, we have done a full structural optimization at the AM1 semiempirical level [4] for a variety of related hard and soft compounds. The optimized structures of dexamethasone (*32*), betamethasone 17α-valerate (*33*), clobetasol 17α-propionate (*3*), hydrocortisone 17α-butyrate (*34*) and triamcinolone acetonide (*35*) indicate that in the critical position of the 21 carbon a heteroatom is exposed in the β-side of the molecule, and probably this is critical for interaction of this pharmacophore with the receptor. A simple cortienic acid methyl ester 17α-carbonate does not have the same exposed heteroatom in the β-position, and it is clearly completely void of any activity. It was found that the chloroethylidine derivative (like *12*) has the preferential conformation with the chlorine atom pointing towards the α-side [5], that is, towards the carbonate moiety. It is 'hid-

Table 1. Binding of selected soft glucocorticoids to the glucocorticoid receptor of rat lung

No.	R_1	R_2	X_1	X_2	X_3	RBA[a]
9	i-C_3H_7	α-CH_3	Cl	F	H	560
10	n-C_3H_7	α-CH_3	Cl	F	H	870
11	n-C_5H_{11}	α-CH_3	Cl	F	H	840
12	i-C_3H_7	β-CH_3	-CH-Cl[c] CH$_3$	H	F	11
13	C_2H_5	α-CH_3	CH_2Cl	F	H	19
14	C_2H_5	α-CH_3	Cl	F	H	740
15[b]	C_2H_5	α-CH_3	Cl	F	H	16
16	i-C_3H_7	α-CH_3	Cl	F	F	1,100
17	n-C_3H_7	α-CH_3	Cl	F	F	1,000
18	n-C_3H_7	α-CH_3	Cl	H	F	1,000
19	CH_3	α-CH_3	Cl	H	F	1,200
20	CH_3	β-CH_3	Cl	F	H	990
21	n-C_3H_7	β-CH_3	Cl	F	H	1,460
22	i-C_3H_7	α-CH_3	F	F	H	820
23	n-C_3H_7	α-CH_3	F	F	H	990
24	C_2H_5	H	F	H	H	200
25	i-C_3H_7	H	F	H	H	70
26	C_2H_5	α-CH_3	Cl	F	F	2,100
27	CH_3	H	Cl	H	H	180
28	C_2H_5	H	Cl	H	H	490
29	n-C_3H_7	H	Cl	H	H	540
30	H^3	β-CH_3	Cl	H	H	3
31	H^3	α-CH_3	Cl	F	H	7

[a] $RBA_{dexamethasone} = 100$.
[b] 11-keto.
[c] Note branching: $\left(\text{COOCH} \begin{smallmatrix} \diagup CH_3 \\ \diagdown Cl \end{smallmatrix} \right)$

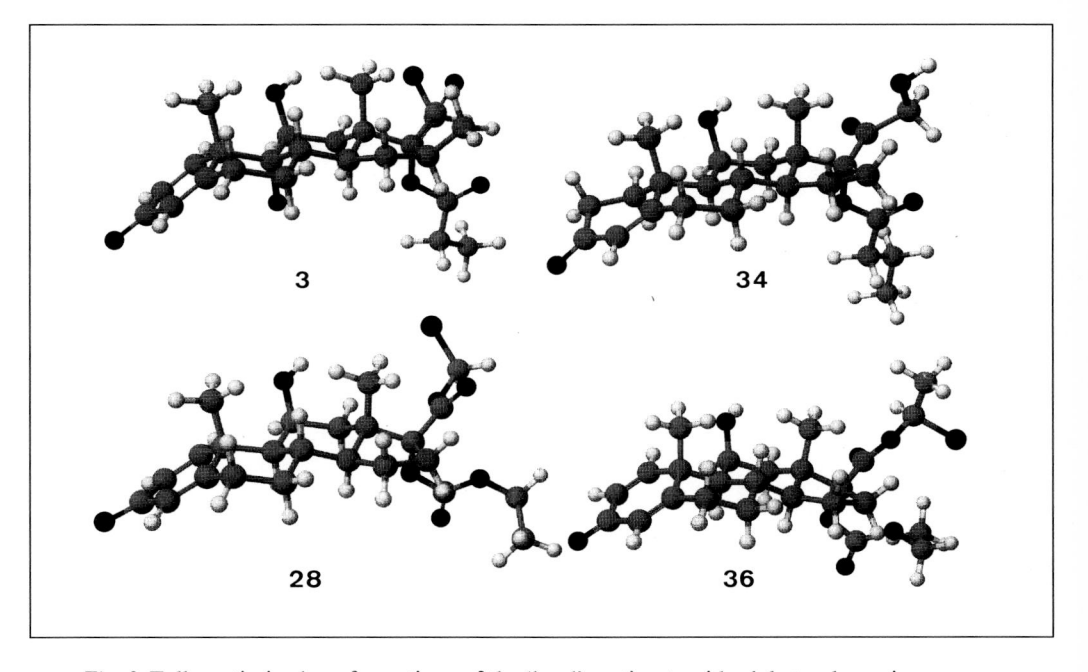

Fig. 3. Fully optimized conformations of the 'hard' corticosteroids clobetasol propionate (*3*), hydrocortisone 17α-butyrate (*34*), the soft steroid loteprednol etabonate (*28*) and its C-α-methyl analog (*36*).

den', and what is exposed to the β-position is the methyl function. This conformation is consistent with the finding that this compound has very weak activity. Calculations of the rotational barrier, that is, to expose the chlorine in the expected 'right' position, would involve 8–10 kcal/mol, that is, a very energy-consuming process, and this is again consistent with the observed very weak activity. On the other hand, the chloromethyl ester, as shown in figure 3, has a chlorine function exposed in a very prominent position in the β-side similar to clobetasol, and this would allow a good interaction at the receptor site of this electronegative function. While all this is suggestive, the whole picture is fully consistent with the need for a heteroatom of the type of oxygen or halogen exposed available in the 21 and/or isoteric position of the molecule.

One of these chloromethyl esters, Δ^1-17α-ethyl carbonate derivative *28,* is being successfully developed for use as a potent and very safe topical steroid. This compound, named loteprednol etabonate, indeed shows significant improvement in the therapeutic index as reflected by the antigranuloma versus thymolytic activity. The value for its therapeutic index (TI = 24) is compared to that of around 1 for clobetasol proprinate, betamethasone valerate or hydrocortisone 17α-butyrate [5]. The close values of the therapeutic indices of these hard steroids support the idea that increasing the intrinsic activity even by more than an order of magnitude (clobetasol proprinate) leads to a parallel increase in the toxic side effects, as well. The receptor binding studies of the compound of choice at this point, loteprednol etabonate, clearly indicate its significant activity, which is about 4 times higher than that of dexamethasone, and, again, the predicted and established metabolites, the Δ^1 cortienic acid 17α-ethyl carbonate (the main metabolite) and the Δ^1 cortienic acid, show virtually no receptor binding activity.

Topical, that is, dermatological application of loteprednol etabonate showed equivalent vasoconstrictor activity in the McKenzie-Staughton test on humans with betamethasone valerate, while topical application on rats showed significantly reduced thymolytic activity [5]. Even the local side effect, that is, skin atrophy, was significantly lower.

Another major general side effect of corticosteroids is the increase in the intraocular pressure after ophthalmic application. It was recently shown that, as opposed to dexamethasone, loteprednol etabonate shows no effect on the intraocular pressure in rabbits [6]. These results were further confirmed on human subjects. After long-term, frequent application, loteprednol etabonate did not show any significant increase in the intraocular pressure, although it was very effective in controlling various ophthalmic inflammatory diseases [7].

In order to complete the picture, pharmacokinetic-metabolic studies of the soft steroid were performed. The results clearly indicate [8] that after intravenous administration of the loteprednol etabonate, both to rats and dogs, the prime and essentially single metabolite is the Δ^1 cortienic acid 17α-ethyl carbonate which, when injected as such, is eliminated extremely fast with a half-life of around 20 min. Metabolic studies in the eye have also indicated the predicted conversion of the active soft steroid to the inactive metabolite in all compartments of the eye [9].

In conclusion, the application of the inactive metabolite approach to glucocorticoids led to highly potent new, soft steroids with high intrinsic activity and very low toxicity. The significant reduction in toxicity is clearly attributed to the metabolism designed into this class of compounds.

Acknowledgements

I wish to express my sincere appreciation to a number of my collaborators who have made significant contributions to these studies. These include first a number of researchers at Otsuka Pharmaceutical Company: Drs. A. Sonoda, S. Tamada, S. Teramoto, S. Nakatsu, M. Honma, M. Kato, T. Morita and Y. Ishisue. They have done most of the synthetic work and preliminary pharmacological evaluations. Some of the pharmacokinetic-metabolic evaluation, particularly of the loteprednol etabonate, were done by Drs. T. Loftsson, W. Wu, H. Derendorf and G. Hochhaus. The receptor binding studies of most of the new soft steroids were done by R. Hochhaus and E. Brunt under the guidance of Dr. G. Hochhaus. Dr. M. Huang contributed to the AM1 study of the conformational relations in hard and soft corticosteroids.

References

1   Bodor N: New methods of drug targeting; in Sardel S, Mechoulam R, Agranat I (eds): Trends in Medicinal Chemistry '90. Oxford, Blackwell, 1992, pp 35–44.
2   Bodor N: The application of soft drug approaches to the design of safer corticosteroids; in Christophers E (ed): Topical Corticosteroid Therapy: A Novel Approach to Safer Drugs. New York, Raven Press, 1988, pp 13–25.
3   Rohdewald P, Moellmann H, Hochhaus G: Receptor binding affinity of commercial glucocorticoids to the glucocorticoid receptor of human lung. Atemwegs Lungenkr 1984;10:484–489.
4   Dewar MJS, Zoebisch EG, Nealy EF, Stewart JJP: AM1, a new general purpose quantum mechanical molecular model. J Am Chem Soc 1985;107:3902–3909.
5   Bodor N: Designing safer ophthalmic drugs; in van der Goot H, Domany G, Pallos L, Timmerman H (eds): Trends in Medicinal Chemistry '88. Amsterdam, Elsevier, 1989, pp 145–164.
6   Bodor N, Wu WM: A comparison of intraocular pressure elevating activity of loteprednol etabonate and dexamethasone in rabbits. Curr Eye Res 1992;11:525–530.
7   Laibovitz R, Howes JR, Bartlett JD: Safety evaluation of the intraocular pressure response to loteprednol etabonate in high steroid responders. ARVO Meet, 1992.
8   Bodor N, Loftsson T, Wu WM: Metabolism, distribution and transdermal penetration of a soft corticosteroid, loteprednol etabonate. Curr Eye Res 1992;9:1275–1278.
9   Druzgala P, Wu WM, Bodor N: Ocular absorption and distribution of loteprednol etabonate, a soft steroid in rabbit eyes. Curr Eye Res 1991;10:933–937.

Nicholas Bodor, PhD, DSc, Center for Drug Discovery, PO Box 100497, JHMHC, Gainesville, FL 32610-0497 (USA)

Korting HC, Maibach HI (eds): Topical Glucocorticoids with Increased Benefit/Risk Ratio.
Curr Probl Dermatol. Basel, Karger, 1993, vol 21, pp 20–28

....

Glucocorticoid Receptors

Maria Ponec

Department of Dermatology, University Hospital Leiden, The Netherlands

Great progress has been made in the last 25 years in understanding the mechanism of glucocorticoid action. It is now generally accepted that most of the actions of glucocorticoids are mediated at the cellular level through an intracellular receptor called the glucocorticoid receptor [reviewed recently in ref. 1–5]. The presence of glucocorticoid receptors has been established in almost all tissues, including cells of the skin [6, 7]. A few actions are mediated through the mineralocorticoid receptor, that mediates the action of aldosterone and other mineralocorticoid hormones [1].

The current model of glucocorticoid action is illustrated in figure 1. The glucocorticoid, G, enters the cell by passive diffusion and binds there specifically and with high affinity to the receptor, R, to form a nonactivated complex GR. The interaction between the receptor and its ligand results in activation or transformation of the glucocorticoid-receptor complex into a DNA-binding protein, GR′. This activation involves dissociation of a large multiprotein complex consisting of one hormone-binding protein, two non-hormone-binding heat shock proteins of 90 kDa, Hsp90, and probably an additional 59-kDa protein that binds directly to Hsp90. Upon binding to specific regions of DNA – the so-called glucocorticoid-responsive elements, GREs [8] – the initiation of the transcription of DNA into RNA takes place. The changes in mRNA levels result in changes in the production of proteins translated by these RNAs. Immunohistochemical staining revealed that in the absence of ligand the R is mostly (but not exclusively) present in the cytosol. Upon ligand binding, the GR complex is localized primarily in the nucleus [9].

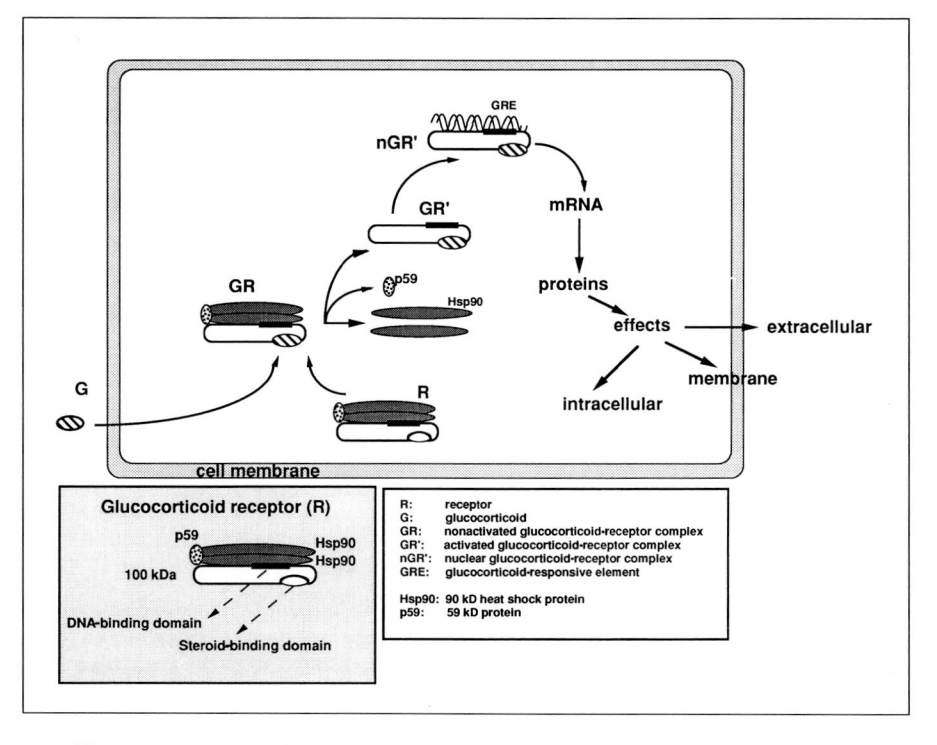

Fig. 1. Receptor-mediated mechanism of glucocorticoid action. See text for explanation.

Structure and Activation of the Glucocorticoid Receptor

The glucocorticoid receptor belongs to a large family of steroid receptors that includes glucocorticoid, estrogen, progesterone, vitamin D, mineralocorticoid, androgen, thyroid and retinoic acid receptors [10, 11]. All these receptors contain three major domains: a ligand-binding, a DNA-binding and a modulatory domain. While the steroid-binding domains possess amino acid sequences that differ widely between different classes of steroids, the DNA-binding domains show a high extent of homology. The size and amino acid composition of the modulatory domain differ at most among various steroid receptors.

The glucocorticoid receptor is a glycoprotein consisting of about 780 amino acids in which the modulatory domain represents the amino-terminal half of the receptor (about 430 amino acids), the centrally located DNA-binding domain contains about 70 amino acids and the adjacent steroid-binding domain that is

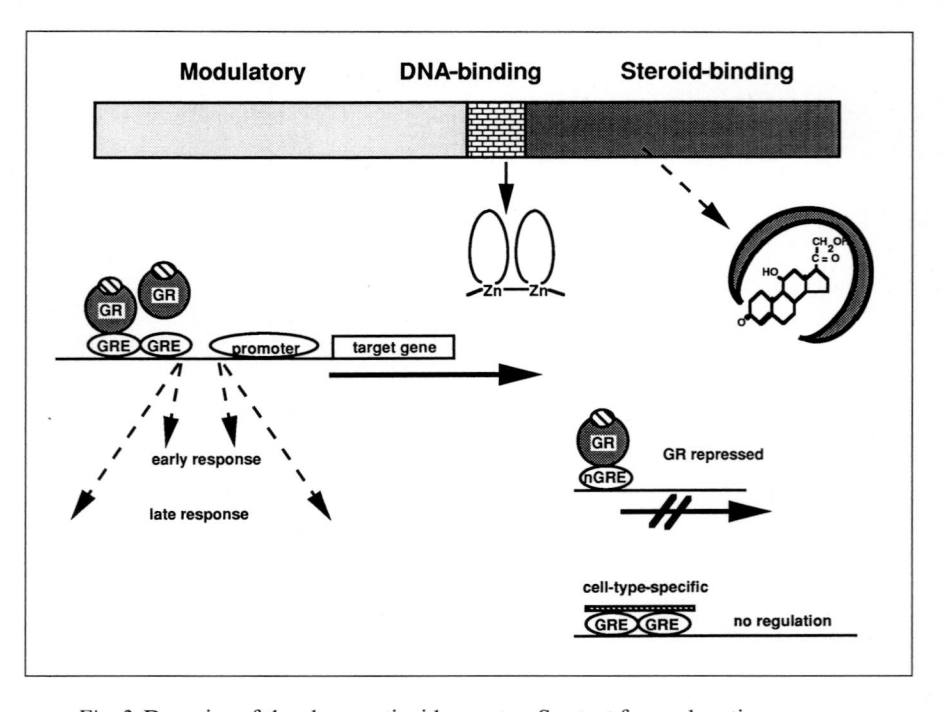

Fig. 2. Domains of the glucocorticoid receptor. See text for explanation.

located at the carboxy terminus occupies about one third of the molecule (fig. 2) [reviewed in ref. 1–5].

The DNA-binding domain is rich in cysteine, lysine and arginine and consists of two repeat units of 25 amino acids each. It has been suggested that each of the repeat sequences could fold into a loop or finger structure similar to Zn-containing loops. This domain has been shown to be capable to bind specifically and with high affinity to GREs. In the absence of ligand, the steroid-binding protein receptor is associated with two Hsp90 proteins that cover in a certain way the DNA-binding domain. The binding of steroid induces a conformational change in the receptors (activation), that results in the dissociation of the heat shock proteins. The activated steroid-receptor complex then binds to DNA and quickly scans the double helix for GRE. The steroid-receptor complex will find target genes with a high GRE content first, resulting in a rapid response to steroid administration. The time course and the magnitude of the hormone response will depend next to the number of GREs also on the affinity of the steroid-receptor complex for GRE and on the distance of GREs from the transcription start site.

When GREs are located far upstream (or downstream) of the promoter, target genes are activated only after several hours of hormone treatment.

The modulatory domain, that reacts with most antireceptor antibodies, contains sequences that amplify the transcriptional regulatory activity. The exact mechanism by which this enhancement occurs is not known, but it is thought to be related to the acidic amino acid composition in this region. Mutations in this domain diminish the receptor activity, but deletion of this region of the receptor does not abolish the ability of the receptor to regulate transcription.

As a result of glucocorticoid administration either induction or repression of target genes may occur, resulting e.g. in enhanced cell proliferation and differentiation or inhibition of cytokine production. In the case of glucocorticoid-induced target gene repression, as for example of urokinase, collagenase or stromelysin genes, this may be a result of the binding of the steroid-receptor complex to 'negative' (nGRE) response sequences. The nGRE consensus sequence differs from the positive one. Different cell types can respond differently to the administration of the same glucocorticoid. For example, the regulation of phosphoenol pyruvate carboxykinase gene expression is positively regulated in kidney cells but negatively regulated in adipose tissue [12]. The tissue-specific glucocorticoid responses are probably not caused by differences in the GRE consensus or in the glucocorticoid-receptor structure, but are most likely a result of a multihormonal regulation that may be cell-specific.

Based on the finding that for optimal steroid binding the presence of amino acids (cysteine and methionine) that are distant from each other in the linear sequence is necessary, a model has been proposed in which the steroid-binding domain is folded to give such a tertiary structure that a hydrophobic pocket is formed that comprises the steroid-binding site. The hormone-binding site exerts a regulatory function, since in the absence of hormone the hormone-binding domain is able to inactivate the receptor even if the receptor is present in the nucleus. Receptors lacking the hormone-binding domain are constitutively functional and located in the nucleus.

Glucocorticoids and Cultured Epidermal Keratinocytes

Specific Intracellular Binding and Structure-Activity Relationship
Since the introduction of cortisone for the treatment of rheumatic arthritis and of hydrocortisone for topical treatment of dermatological diseases more than 40 years ago, a great number of synthetic analogues of hydrocortisone have been produced and used to suppress inflammatory and immunological responses in various dermatological disorders. Most of the synthetic steroid derivatives showed higher clinical efficacy than hydrocortisone did. One of the factors affect-

Table 1. Structure and molecular manipulations of hydrocortisone

Ring	Modification	Derivative (examples)	Relative binding affinity[a]
A	1–2 double bond	prednisolone	2.2
B	9α-fluorination	9α-fluorohydrocortisone	2.9
		9α-fluoroprednisolone	2.9
C	C_{11} oxygen	cortisone	no binding
D	16β-methylation	betamethasone	2.2
	16β-hydroxylation	triamcinolone	1.7
	16,17-acetonide	triamcinolone acetonide	4.6
	17-esterification	hydrocortisone 17-butyrate	3.6
		betamethasone 17-valerate	13.0
		clobetasol 17-propionate	8.0
	21-esterification	hydrocortisone 21-acetate	0.1
		betamethasone 21-valerate	1.4
	17,21-diesterification	betamethasone 17,21-divalerate	4.8
	21-chlorination	clobetasol	6.8
		clobetasol 17-propionate	8.1

[a] Data are given as ratio of IC_{50} values of hydrocortisone and the steroid derivative [modified from ref. 7 and 13–15], where IC_{50} is the concentration of a steroid derivative necessary to displace 50% of ^{3}H-dexamethasone from the receptor.

ing the biological effect is the affinity by which the steroid binds to the glucocorticoid receptor. In table 1, the major molecular modifications of the hydrocortisone structure and the effects of these modifications on the affinity to the receptor are presented. The results of the binding studies performed with isolated cytosol fractions of cultured human skin epidermal keratinocytes showed in which way a substituent on the steroid molecule can affect the binding affinity of the steroid

Table 2. Structure and molecular manipulations of cortisone

Ring	Modification	Derivative (examples)	Relative binding affinity[a]
A	1–2 double bond	prednisone	no binding
B	9α-fluorination	9α-fluorocortisone	0.2
		9α-fluoroprednisone	0.2
D	21-chlorination	clobetasone	5.6
	17-esterification	clobetasone 17-butyrate	10.0

[a] Data are given as ratio of IC_{50} values of hydrocortisone and the steroid derivative [modified from ref. 7 and 13–15], where IC_{50} is the concentration of a steroid derivative necessary to displace 50% of ^{3}H-dexamethasone from the receptor.

for the glucocorticoid receptor [13–15]. It became clear that the presence of an olefinic bond between C-1 and C-2, a fluorine atom at the 9α position, a hydroxyl group at the 11β position and an ester group at the 17α position all of them increase the affinity of the steroid for the receptor. On the other hand, esterification of the hydroxyl group at C-21 leads to a decrease in the affinity of the steroid for the receptor. Quite remarkable was the finding that a steroid derivative possessing a keto group at the 11β position – clobetasone 17-butyrate – showed relatively high affinity for the receptor, while prednisone, from which it was derived, did not bind to the receptor at all. The structure-binding studies revealed that the presence of a fluorine atom at the 9α position as in 9α-F-cortisone could partially counteract the negative effect of this keto group. Furthermore, the affinity for the receptor increased by introducing a chlorine atom at the 21 position and by the introduction of an ester group at the 17α position (table 2).

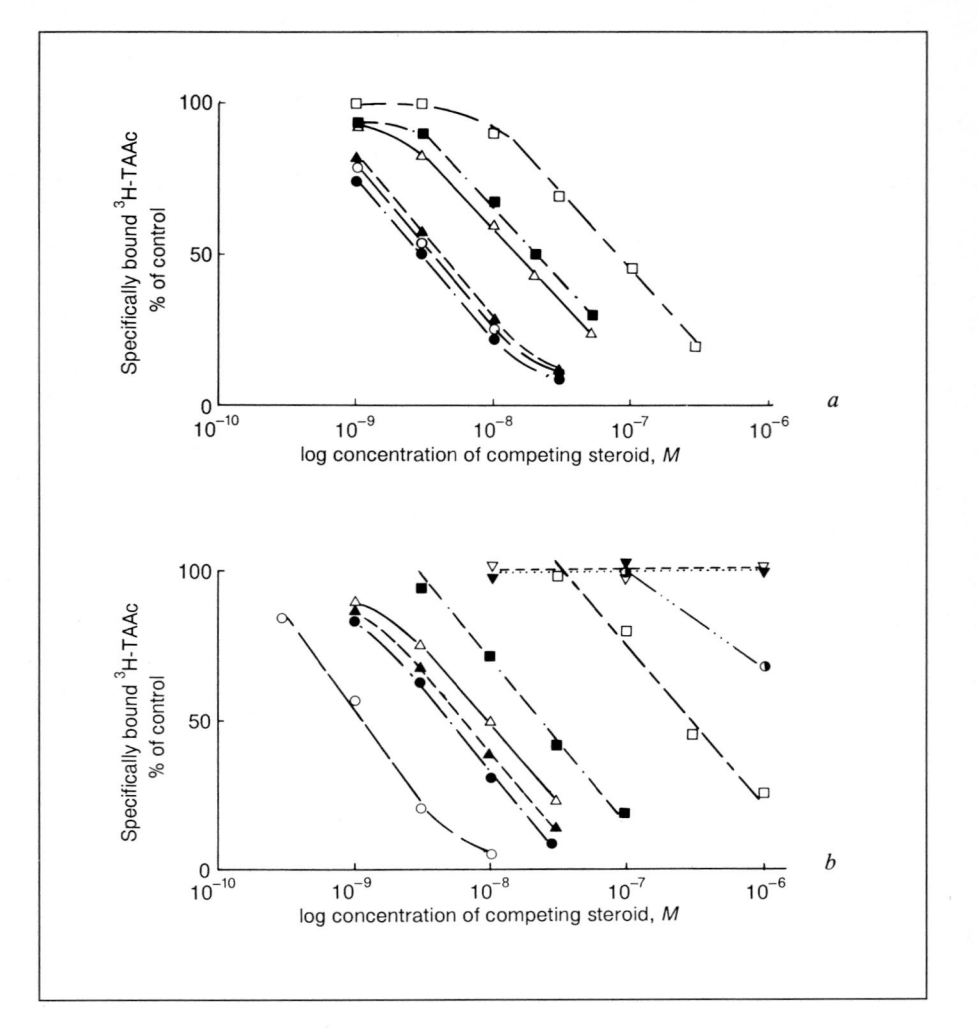

Fig. 3. Displacement of bound ^{3}H-triamcinolone acetonide (TAAc) by various unlabeled steroid derivatives measured in cell-free cytosol (*a*) and whole-cell receptor binding assay (*b*). Aliquots of cytosol fraction (*a*) or confluent keratinocyte cultures (*b*) were incubated overnight at $0\,^{\circ}C$ (*a*) or for 4 h at $37\,^{\circ}C$ (*b*) with $10^{-8}\,M$ ^{3}H-TAAC in the presence of increasing concentrations of nonlabeled steroids, and the competition for specific binding was measured, as described earlier [6]. Binding in the absence of any competing steroid is expressed as 100%, and the results are plotted as a percentage of this binding. The specificity of glucocorticoid-receptor binding is demonstrated by low-extent binding of progesterone and absence of binding of 17β-estradiol and nandrolone. □ = Hydrocortisone; △ = triamcinolone acetonide; ● = betamethasone 17-valerate; ◐ = progesterone; ▽ = 17β-estradiol; ■ = hydrocortisone 17-butyrate; ▲ = clobetasone 17-butyrate; ○ = clobetasol 17-propionate; ▼ = nandrolone.

Cellular Uptake

The final effect of a glucocorticoid will not only depend on its binding affinity to the glucocorticoid receptor, but also on the amount of glucocorticoid reaching the target cells. In the case glucocorticoid is applied in a topical dermatological preparation, the amount reaching the cell will be determined by its diffusion rate through the stratum corneum, which will depend next to the composition of the formulation also on the steroid structure. Once reaching the viable cells of the epidermis and the dermis, the cellular uptake and the duration of the steroid stay within the cell will determine its final clinical efficacy. From studies with cultured human fibroblasts and keratinocytes it became clear that the cellular uptake and the duration of its stay within the cell strongly depend on physicochemical properties of the steroid derivative [16]. In the whole-cell glucocorticoid receptor binding study which is performed with whole cells by combining the receptor binding and the steroid cellular uptake, a very good correlation can be obtained between steroid-binding potency and its clinical efficacy (fig. 3).

Conclusion

The final therapeutic effect of a topically applied glucocorticoid will depend on a number of processes that take place after its administration: (1) on the rate of penetration through and the duration of its stay within the stratum corneum; (2) on the cellular uptake and the affinity of the glucocorticoid receptor for a particular steroid; (3) on the rate of its metabolic biotransformation within the skin which may lead to the steroid inactivation, and last but not least (4) on processes that take place after the steroid binding to the receptor. These processes include (a) the rate of turnover of the various glucocorticoid-regulated mRNAs and their protein products, (b) the delay time of the initiation of macromolecular synthesis that is a cause of a lag time of several hours before the effect of steroid is evident, (c) the duration of the responses that can last for some time after the tissue levels of steroid drop, and (d) on the rate the steroid is cleared from the tissue. The rate of the latter process may vary between the individuals and can be affected by the disease. The knowledge of all the above-mentioned steps can help in designing the frequency of the treatment which may be once or several times during the day or on alternative days.

References

1 Munck A, Mendel DB, Smith LI, Orti E: Glucocorticoid receptors and action. Am Rev Respir Dis 1990;141:S2–S10.
2 Pratt WB: Glucocorticoid receptor structure and the initial events in signal transduction. Molecular Endocrinology and Steroid Action. Prog Clin Biol Res 1990;322:119–132.

3 Baxter JD: Minimizing the side-effects of glucocorticoid therapy. Adv Intern Med 1990;35:173–194.

4 Gustafsson JA, Carlstedt-Duke J, Strömstedt PE, Wikström AC, Denis M, Okret S, Dong Y: Structure, function and regulation of the glucocorticoid receptor. Molecular Endocrinology and Steroid Action. Prog Clin Biol Res 1990;322:65–80.

5 Godowski PJ, Picard D: Steroid receptors: How to be both receptor and transcription factor. Biochem Pharmacol 1989;38:3135–3143.

6 Ponec M, de Kloet ER, Kempenaar JA: Corticoids and cultured human skin fibroblasts: Intracellular specific binding in relation to growth inhibition. J Invest Dermatol 1980;75:293–296.

7 Ponec M, Kempenaar JA, de Kloet ER: Corticoids and cultured human epidermal keratinocytes: Specific intracellular binding and clinical efficacy. J Invest Dermatol 1981;76:211–214.

8 Yamamoto KR: Steroid receptor regulated transcription of specific genes and networks. Annu Rev Genet 1985;19:209–232.

9 Wikström AC, Bakke O, Okret S, Bronnegard M, Gustafsson J: Intracellular localization of the glucocorticoid receptor: Evidence for cytoplasmic and nuclear localization. Endocrinology 1987;120:1232–1239.

10 Evans RM: The steroid action and thyroid hormone receptor superfamily. Science 1988;240:889–895.

11 Green S, Chambon P: Nuclear receptors enhance our understanding of transcription regulation. Trends Genet 1988;4:191–217.

12 Nechushtan H, Benvenisty N, Brandeus R, Reshef L: Glucocorticoids control phosphoenolpyruvate carboxykinase gene expression in a tissue specific manner. Nucleic Acids Res 1987;15:6407–6417.

13 Ponec M: Glucocorticoids and cultured human skin cells: Specific intracellular binding and structure-activity relationship. Br J Dermatol 1982;107(suppl 23):24–29.

14 Shroot B, Caron JC, Ponec M: Glucocorticoid specific binding: Structure-activity relationships. Br J Dermatol 1982;107(suppl 23):30–34.

15 Ponec M, Kempenaar J, Shroot B, Caron JC: Glucocorticoids: Binding affinity and lipophilicity. J Pharm Sci 1986;75:973–975.

16 Ponec M, Kempenaar JA: Biphasic entry of glucocorticoids into cultured human skin keratinocytes and fibroblasts. Arch Dermatol Res 1983;275:334–344.

Maria Ponec, PhD, Department of Dermatology, Bldg. 16, University Hospital, PO Box 9600, NL–2300 RC Leiden (The Netherlands)

Korting HC, Maibach HI (eds): Topical Glucocorticoids with Increased Benefit/Risk Ratio.
Curr Probl Dermatol. Basel, Karger, 1993, vol 21, pp 29–44

....

Methods of Computer-Aided Drug Design and Their Applications to Steroids

Terry R. Stouch

Bristol-Myers Squibb Pharmaceutical Research Institute, Princeton, N.J., USA

The field of computational chemistry comprises a large number of diverse methods for studying chemical problems computationally. Many of the methods of computational chemistry have proven useful in the study of biologically active compounds, and 'computer-aided drug design' (CADD) is now a well-established tool in most pharmaceutical companies [1, 2]. These methods are valuable aids in determining, understanding and comparing the structures and properties of small, drug-sized molecules. They also assist the study of the large biomolecule targets of drugs. Methods have been proposed for use in essentially all of the stages of a drug discovery and development program, including lead discovery, lead optimization and toxicity testing. Studies of drug 'design' fall into two general classes, those that try to derive the requirements of the target from the structures and already-known biological activities of a number of compounds, and those that utilize the atomic-level structures of the protein targets.

Steroids have been the subject of many computational studies for over 2 decades. Their important role in physiology, their well-defined structures and reasonably rigid geometry, and the mass of available biological information have, in fact, made some of them almost standard sets of data with which to investigate new computational methods. This paper consists of two parts. In the second part, a number of these studies are reviewed. However, since the plethora of available methods and their application can be confusing and difficult to follow, and since many different methods will be discussed in the review of applications to steroids, the first part will consist of an introduction to the methods and techniques of CADD with an emphasis on those methods applied to steroids in part II.

In the limited space of this paper, it is impossible to give anything but a brief overview of this large and burgeoning field. Luckily, a number of high-quality introductions and reviews of the specific topics are available, and these comprise the emphasis of the references.

Part I: Methods of Computational Chemistry

Computer Graphics

Interactive computer graphics is now a standard tool of the computational chemist. The three-dimensional, visual natural of the fields of chemistry, biochemistry and biology requires real-time interaction with three-dimensional representations of both small drug molecules and large protein structures. Most commercially available molecular modeling programs are now closely integrated with computer graphics that run on a range of devices from fairly inexpensive personal computers through midrange workstations costing from US $10,000 to 50,000, to workstations costing much more. Thanks to the computing revolution, most graphical displays now come as part of a workstation environment rather than stand-alone graphical devices that must be interfaced with a computer, such as was common in the past. The relatively low cost and impressive power of even inexpensive workstations make them a common tool for the practicing computational chemist.

Color graphics, smooth, real-time rotation of molecules, a variety of different types of molecular displays (stick drawings, CPK representations, various surface representations), superposition of a number of molecules at one time, the ability to quickly build new molecules and access databases of molecules, and seamless interfaces to molecular mechanics and quantum mechanics programs are features that experienced users now expect of computer graphics programs. Even moderately priced workstations will allow the display and real-time interaction with proteins of many thousands of atoms and rapid determinations of accurate three-dimensional structures of small molecules. These platforms are indispensable to efficient computational studies and relieve much of the drudgery that, until recently, was a time-consuming part of this work.

Molecular Modeling and Three-Dimensional Molecular Structures

The three-dimensional nature of molecular shape and structure is a central theme in most drug design studies. The concept of the 'lock and key' fit between the shapes of the drug ligands and their target proteins is central to most drug design projects, even those that proceed without the benefit of the structure of the target proteins. For molecules of any complexity, an understanding of the three-dimensional relationships between a series of drug molecules or between a drug and the protein must start with the three-dimensional coordinates of a molecule's atoms.

Physical models have been of great use to chemists, and computer-generated models prove to be even more useful. The right software usually makes building molecules on the computer easier than by hand, especially if models are required for many molecules. Computer models are always as accurate as physical models and can be much more so. In addition, many molecules can be compared, superimposed and manipulated at one time, tasks impossible for physical models. Also, they can be docked into a similar representation of a receptor binding site or enzyme active site. Using computer graphics, molecules can be visualized in many ways. And last, they serve as a starting point for calculation of a number of other properties such as molecular volume, surface area, other conformations, energies and, when coupled with quantum mechanics, electronic properties.

Molecular Mechanics. A number of programs are available for generating models with idealized geometry at a 'wire-model' level of approximation either from a sketch of the molecule on a computer screen or by linking together three-dimensional molecular fragments. These models usually have an 'idealized' geometry where bond lengths and angles assume some standard, average values. For a study of any detail, however, this level of approximation is often insufficient and usually more accurate models are generated, often using molecular mechanics [3–6]. The molecular mechanics formalism treats a molecule as bonded atoms, and a 'strain' energy is calculated as a function of the deviation of structural features from 'optimum' values and the energy penalties exacted by those deviations. The features are usually bond lengths, angles between 2 consecutive bonds and 'torsional' or dihedral angles representing the degree of rotation about single bonds. Other terms are also usually included, in particular van der Waals and electrostatic interactions. The form of this function is referred to as the 'potential energy function', and the optimum values and energy penalties are referred to as the parameters of the function. Together they are often referred to as 'force fields'. In essence, a particular molecular model is dissembled into its components bonds, angles, torsions and interatomic interactions. The values of the components are calculated, compared to their optimum values, and the energy penalties for any deviations are summed to provide the strain energy. To this value is added the energy of the interatomic interactions to provide the total potential energy of the molecule.

This is a simplified view of the force fields whose functional forms can be quite detailed and complicated and whose parameterization can become very specific. Using such force fields, impressive accuracy can be achieved in the prediction of subtleties of molecular geometries and energies, energies of rotational barriers, and vibrational frequencies. However, force field development and parameterization can be difficult, time-consuming and thankless tasks [7, 8]. The more complicated and highly parameterized force fields become, the fewer the molecules to which they can be applied.

The force field provides the potential energy 'surface' of the molecule. As the geometry of the molecule changes, i.e. as the atoms are moved relative to each other, different parts of the surface will be sampled. Energy minimization (or geometry optimization) algorithms search the surface for low-energy arrangements of the atoms. Also, parts of the energy surface can be selectively searched to probe the energies of interconversions between different molecular conformations. Additionally, the derivative of the potential energy with respect to the atomic coordinates provides the force on each atom. Using Newton's equations of motions, these forces can be used to calculate the positions and velocities of the atoms over time. This is the basis of molecular dynamics simulations which are used to study molecular motions, to sample different molecular conformations, and in structure determination using X-ray crystallographic or nuclear magnetic resonance (NMR) data [9–11].

Quantum Mechanics. Quantum mechanics is also used to generate three-dimensional molecular structures through the application of approximations to the solution of Schroedinger's equation [3, 12, 13]. Like molecular mechanics, energies are calculated for any particular interatomic arrangement and so a potential energy surface is defined. However, whereas molecular mechanics determines the energy of a particular arrangement of atoms from a predefined set of atomic bonds and a potential energy function and typically ignores the electrons within the molecule, quantum mechanical methods typically deal only with the electronic configurations and energies are calculated from something approaching first principals as applied to the electronic configuration of a specific atomic arrangement. Quantum mechanical methods are more powerful than molecular mechanics in that, in addition to molecular geometry, electronic properties can be calculated, excited states can be addressed and reaction pathways can be studied. In addition, these methods require little of the parameterization required of molecular mechanics and so they can be applied to a much wider range of molecules. Unfortunately, the disadvantage of these methods is that they are extremely time-consuming. For similar accuracy of molecular geometry, quantum mechanical methods can easily take thousands or tens-of-thousands of times more computer time than does molecular mechanics. Tasks of seconds for molecular mechanics might require hours, days or weeks for quantum mechanical methods.

Quantum mechanical methods are divided into two camps, semiempirical methods and ab initio methods. The former are less rigorous, require parameterization (but much less so than do molecular mechanics) and are conceptually more limited than the latter; however, they take much less time than ab initio methods and, for many classes of molecules, provide quite reasonable results.

Conformational Search. Most biological molecules have more than one conformer accessible to them at normal room temperature; however, geometry optimization methods provide only one at a time. Except for special cases, the conformation responsible for eliciting a biological effect is seldom obvious and an

---

entire field has developed around the enumeration and sampling of possible conformers. Simple arithmetic shows the potential enormity of the task. A small molecule can easily have 6 rotatable bonds. If we assume that individual conformers can be defined within a 30° tolerance (not a small value), there would be 360/30 = 12 possible conformers about each bond or a total of 12^6 or 3 million conformers. If the act of generating, optimizing and evaluating the energy of each conformer consumed just 1 s, the task of enumerating these conformers would require 830 h of computer time for this one small molecule, alone. Often dozens or hundreds of molecules must be investigated. A number of methods have been applied to this problem and conformational search algorithms have been the centerpieces of several programs [14–16].

Other Methods. In addition to the methods mentioned above, some programs are available that allow very rapid generation of reasonable three-dimensional structures from two-dimensional structures. The results of these methods are approximate; however, their speed allows them to be applied to large numbers of compounds in a reasonable amount of time and they have been of considerable use for large databases of hundreds of thousands of two-dimensional structures [17].

Database Search

Searching for two- or three-dimensional structures in large chemical databases has been an active area of research [18, 19]. Many such large databases of chemical structures, properties and biological activities have been assembled over the years privately, publicly and commercially. They contain a potential wealth of information that has, until recently, been difficult to exploit. However, the promise of effective searches for assisting drug discovery has warrented a considerable effort in this area by many groups and software companies. Molecular structural data tend to be somewhat unique, and specialized programs have been developed for their storage and retrieval.

In general, two different types of searches can be done: two-dimensional and three-dimensional. Two-dimensional searches use queries concerning a molecule's constituent elements and atom-atom connectivities, the chemical graph, without any consideration of the three-dimensional spatial arrangement of the atoms. Such searches are useful for locating a specific compound, or compounds containing particular functional groups or skeletal backbones, such as the 5-ring steroid nucleus.

Three-dimensional searches are considerably more ambitious and potentially even more rewarding. These methods search for particular three-dimensional arrangements of atoms, such as a suspected 'pharmacophore', the required arrangement of bulk, hydrophobicity, charged groups and hydrogen-bonding responsible for a molecule's biological activity. The definition of a pharmacophore, coupled with three-dimensional database search, makes possible the discovery of compounds with similar biological activity, but yet only the minimum necessary structural relationship. This promises more rapid discovery of small organic molecules that mimic the activity of larger biological molecules. Also, compounds with similar biological activities yet very different profiles otherwise might be discovered. Finally, this could provide a means of obtaining desired activity while avoiding the claims of active patents.

Chemical Property Prediction

The prediction of the properties of molecules has been a key use of computational chemistry. Many properties can be successfully calculated using a variety of techniques for a wide range of compounds. This is advantageous when experimentally determined values are difficult, expensive or impossible to obtain, such as when a compound does not exist. These properties include, in addition to the geometries and energies inherent in molecular models: heats of formation; dipole moments; pK_as; vibrational frequencies and intensities; solubility; molecular volume, surface area and shape; measures of molecular complexity and topology; boiling points; electrostatic fields; molar refractivity; hydrogen-bonding propensities; polarizabilities, and others. Boyd [20] provides a fairly exhaustive list.

Structure-Activity Relationships

Ultimately, in a drug design study, the results of the molecular mechanics, quantum mechanics, database searches and property calculation are applied to rationalizing the relationship between a molecule's structure (or, more generally, its properties, including the property of structure) and its biological activity [21–23]. A great number of approaches to assist this rationalization process have been suggested, and each has its strengths and weaknesses. This section will discuss methods for the derivation of such relationships without benefit of the three-dimensional atomic structure of the target protein. These methods use the structures and known biological activities of a number of compounds to determine the particular features and properties that are responsible for eliciting the biological effect. They are often lumped in the category of 'QSAR' (quantitative structure-activity relationships), because in many cases they developed as extensions to earlier QSAR (linear free energy) approaches [24].

The features and properties that have been related to bioactivity are many and diverse. Perhaps the best known and earliest methods used a Hammett-type linear free-energy approach ('Hansch' analysis) to relate measured physical properties of substituents (e.g. electron donating and withdrawing capacity, steric bulk) to biological activity. Calculated and measured indices of lipophilicity, indices of molecular complexity and topology, substructural fragments, molecular volume, molecular surface area, atomic partial charges, molecular shape and the shapes of substituents, and electrostatic fields are some of the molecular features that have been related to activity.

Typically, these methods use multivariate analysis (such as multiple regression, pattern recognition, cluster analysis or statistical methods) to find and evaluate a relationship between these features and the activities. Once such a relationship is established, it can be used to predict the activity of new, potentially even hypothetical, molecules and often can be used to understand the mechanism of activity.

Often, these studies are performed on series of analogues with identical structural backbones (such as the steroid nucleus) with variation restricted to changes at common sites of substitution. These studies do not explicitly consider the conformation, and the implicit assumption is that all compounds of the series have similar conformational properties or that conformational fluctuations will not alter the particular activity in question (these are not always good assumptions). Often such studies are useful for 'fine-tuning' the substitution pattern of a particular skeletal framework during the optimization stage of drug design.

The 'active analogue' approach of Marshall and Motoc [25] took the QSAR approach several steps further by explicitly incorporating molecular shape and conformation. Again, the study starts with the structures of a series of compounds with known biological activity. A key feature of this method is that the accessible conformations of the most active molecules are first determined. It is assumed that all compounds with similar activity should be able to achieve some similar conformation(s). The other molecules are evaluated for this capacity and superimposed on the most active compound. The molecular volumes of the superimposed molecules are quantified, and the differences between them are related, using regression methods, to the differences in biological activities.

Cramet et al. [26] also expanded on the more conventional SAR methods with the 'CoMFA' (comparative molecular field analysis) approach. Again a series of molecules of known biological activity are chosen. Prior to the analysis, an active conformation for these molecules is hypothesized, the molecules are placed in that conformation and their three-dimensional structures are superimposed. Using 'probes', steric and electrostatic 'fields' of the molecules are calculated at positions on a three-dimensional grid surrounding the molecules. The values of the fields at the grid points are used as the features of the molecules and are related to the activities using a relatively new analytical method, partial least squares (PLS).

Target-Directed Drug Design

The SAR methods described above address the study of drug action and design from the drug's perspective. However, with the advances in experimental and computational methods [27–29] of determining the macromolecular struc-

---

ture of biomolecules, the three-dimensional atomic-level structure of a number of the protein 'targets' of pharmaceuticals has been determined. This has opened up the field of so-called 'rational' or, perhaps better, targeted drug design. Now drug design can proceed from the other direction. Rather than using the activities of small molecules to attempt to infer the shape and geography of the target, the target can be directly examined, usually using computer graphics.

Unfortunately, contrary to early expectations, the actual design of a small molecule drug, even using knowledge of its site of action, is not straightforward. Protein binding sites and enzymatic active sites are complex affairs. Often they are mobile and the motion of the molecules play a part in biological function. Although molecular dynamics simulation can be employed, its interpretation is not always easy. Further, other factors, such as desolvation and transport, play a role in biochemical processes, issues that protein structures do not address. Finally, it is simply not always a direct process to determine how to best wedge a molecule into a dynamic and sometimes very specific cavity.

Nonetheless, many are trying very hard to do just this, and a number of approaches, techniques and programs have been developed. These methods include the combination of three-dimensional database searching directed by a description of the binding site, definition of the 'potentials' of the binding site to aid in the placement of the functional groups of small molecules, determination of 'best fit' of a putative drug through conformational search of the small molecule within the binding site, strategies for 'docking' rigid molecules in the site, and calculations of binding energies once the molecule is docked [30, 31].

One potentially very powerful approach are methods of calculating differences in free energies of protein-ligand systems based on molecular dynamics or Monte Carlo simulations. Although this method shows promise, it is computationally very intensive, is still developmental and has several pitfalls that place its use best in the hands of experts [32, 33].

An Integrated Approach

The various computational methods are, by no means, mutually exclusive. Often, the difficult task of drug design requires a combination of them in tandem. A single research project might include conformational search coupled with molecular mechanics to dock small molecules into the active site of a protein structure determined, in part, by computational methods of protein structural prediction. This might be followed by three-dimensional database searches that identify novel compounds. Properties of the resulting molecules might then be predicted using quantum mechanics and subsequently included in a QSAR equation. Although earlier studies often dealt with the application or development of individual techniques, as computational chemists and software become more sophisticated, more and more tandem applications of methods occur [34].

Computer-Assisted Drug Design Successes

Although computational methods appear quite powerful, there are certainly instances where they are not as powerful or general as one might want. It is not unfair to ask how and, in fact, whether, computational chemistry actually assists in the day-to-day practice of drug development. The most modest response is that computational chemistry serves as another instrument which provides additional information on molecular structure and properties much as does an NMR or mass spectrometer. Certainly, a testament to this use are the thousands of papers including computations that appear yearly, not only in specialized journals, but also in journals of applied medicinal chemistry, chemistry and agricultural chemistry.

Still, the promise of these methods is greater than that and, in fact, several instances of drug design have been documented. Hansch [35], in a frank review of the field, likens SAR to 'prospecting' for new discoveries and relates how that prospecting has assisted in the development of heart drugs and herbicides. He further describes the development of norfloxacin, an antibiotic, and bromobutamide, a herbicide, whose development were completely attributed to linear free-energy methods of QSAR and which are now commercial products.

Boyd [20] in a more recent review of computation success stories, describes three levels of success. He classifies commercial products, such as those presented by Hansch, as the 'ultimate level of success' and adds two other products to Hansch's list, metamitron and myclobutanil, herbicides designed by QSAR approaches.

Additional Sources of Information

Many of the references provided above will serve as good foothold into the respective fields of study. Computational studies are routinely published in a wide number of journals and no one serves as a central repository. The *Journal of Medicinal Chemistry,* the *Journal of the American Chemical Society,* the *Journal of Computational Chemistry,* the *Journal of Computer-Aided Molecular Design,* the *Journal of Chemical Information and Computer Science,* and *Computers and Chemistry,* all have been repositories of drug design studies and methodology. Recently, the computational chemistry literature has been reviewed [36].

Several books are available that deal with computational chemistry as a whole, drug design or some aspect of computational chemistry [5, 21,22, 37–41].

There are about 10 major software houses that deal largely or wholly in chemistry software. Many academic groups also market their software, usually at a lower price. The Quantum Chemistry Program Exchange [42] has been a valuable repository of software that has been freely contributed by individuals and distributed for a nominal price. Several recent publications provide listings of software and their availability [41, 43, 44].

Part II: Computational Studies of Steroids

As methods of computational chemistry developed over the last several decades, they have often been applied to studies of steroid bioactivity. Linear free-energy methods [45–47], Free-Wilson analysis [48, 49], conformational analysis [50] and quantum mechanics [51] were all used in early studies. More recently, as computational methods matured, more detailed studies have been conducted.

The remainder of this paper constitutes a review of a number of the applications that have been published since 1985. To provide a greater scope, included are studies of a variety of different types and activities of steroids, in addition to topically active glucocorticoids. It is seldom that a particular technique is specific for one type of activity or structural type, and techniques applicable to one class of molecule or one type of activity are often applicable to others, as well.

Bohl and Sussmilch [52] employed the semiempirical quantum mechanical method, CNDO, to determine the three-dimensional structures, charge distribution and molecular electrostatic potential of 2 cardiotonic 2-14β-hydroxylsteroids with nitrogen-containing 17β substituents. They concluded that flexibility of the steroid backbone was of some importance and that there was no electrostatic interaction between the C-20 position and the digitalis receptor. Pasa-Tolic et al. [53] applied ab initio self-consistent field methods of quantum chemistry utilizing a minimal basis set to develop a three-dimensional model of β-androstane and to investigate the possibility of long-range interactions between substituents at the 3 and 16 positions of the steroid nucleus via 'ribbon-like' molecular orbitals.

Bohl [54] used molecular mechanics coupled with conformational search of the 17α-ethyl and 17β side chains of a 17α-ethyl-17β-hydroxyl steroid and found that the preferred conformation of the α substituent might directly affect the ability of the β substituent to interact with a favorable location on the receptor and also might indirectly affect that favorable interaction by modifying the D ring conformation.

Conformational analysis coupled with molecular mechanics was used by Li and Brueggemeier [55] to understand the level of inhibition of steroidal aromatase of a series of 7α-substituted androstenediones. They found that phenyl rings could orient in substantially different ways for phenalkyl substituents than when the phenyl was directly attached at the 7 position and speculated on the resulting possibilities for binding to the enzyme.

Molecular modeling and molecular mechanics were used by White and Breslow [56] to explain experimentally observed template directed chlorinations of steroids as well as the observed conformational restriction of the C_{17}-C_{20} single bond in cholestanol.

Dunn et al. [57], in a study relating measures of molecular surface area with the logarithm of the partition coefficient between hydrophobic solvents and water, had good success at estimating the rate of diffusion of 11 steroids across the stratum corneum.

In efforts to refine methods of database searching and biological activity estimation, Willett and coworkers [58] included a set of steroids in the evaluation of a 'fragment weights' method for estimating bioactivity from analysis of both two- and three-dimensional substructures contained within steroid structures. They used the same data in comparison of methods for determining the similarity of three-dimensional molecular structures [59].

In similar work, Rum and Herndon [60] found high correlations between a molecular similarity measure, calculated from two-dimensional chemical structure graphs, and the affinity to human corticosteroid-binding globin of 47 steroids. They further compared their approach with other methods of structure-activity correlation.

Using pattern recognition methods and a Free-Wilson-type approach to describe molecular structure, Bodor et al. [61] studied the activity of 120 steroids in the McKenzie-Stoughton human vasoconstrictor assay. Stouch and Jurs [62, 63] expanded on that work by utilizing physicochemical parameters, refining the data set, and investigating the SAR using a number of multivariate analytical approaches. They further demonstrated that the results could be used to predict the activities of new compounds with considerable success.

Using linear free-energy Hansch-type analysis, Ebert et al. [64] related physical properties, primarily lipophilicity and size, of a series of 1,3-dioxolane-2-yl-methyltriazoles and 1,3-dioxane-2-yl-methyltriazoles to their in vitro ability to inhibit sterol 14α demethylation and in vitro antifungal activity.

Zeelen [65] provided a detailed review and critique of a substantial number of QSAR and molecular modeling studies of steroids, in particular of a series of cardiac glycosides, and questioned an apparent overreliance on X-ray crystallographic data, the small number of compounds used in several studies, and the frequent underestimation of steroid flexibility.

In the absence of experimentally determined three-dimensional structures of steroid receptor sites, a number of QSAR studies have attempted to use steroid structures and known biological activities to define this site. Simon and Bohl [66] determined a 'hypermolecular' using atomic superpositions of three-dimensional structures from which steric difference and hydrophobic indices were used to define the gestagenic receptor site cavity from the binding affinity data for 55 progesterone derivatives.

This approach has also been used, in addition to molecular mechanics, conformational analysis and quantum chemical methods, to study the role of C_4–C_5 unsaturation in competitive aromatase inhibition. In addition to relating physical properties to biological activity, Bohl et al. [67] found that this unsaturation imposes a conformation favorable to hydroxylation.

As an introduction of the CoMFA method of three-dimensional QSAR, Cramer et al. [26] calculated steric and electrostatic fields for 21 superimposed three-dimensional steroid structures and used the PLS method of multivariate analysis to relate them to the binding constants for corticosteroid- and testosterone-binding globins. This work was expanded on by Kellog et al. [68], who included the use of a 'hydrophobic' field by use of an atom fragment addition approach to calculate hydrophobicity.

Norinder [69] used similar analysis and a molecular lipophilic 'potential' index to develop a three-dimensional QSAR using PLS after conformational analysis of the side chains of 37 steroids assayed for binding to human corticosteroid-binding globin. He extended this work and used difference maps to compare analyses of binding to both human and guinea pig corticosteroid-binding globins and identified regions of the three-dimensional SAR responsible for selectivity [70].

Selectivity was also the subject of a molecular modeling study by Laughton and Neidle [71] who used molecular mechanics and conformational analysis to study the testosterone- and pregnonolone-mimicking conformations of pyridylacetic acid derivatives, and related them to their inhibition of the cytochrome P450 enzymes aromatase and lyase.

Finally, Hui et al. [72] used an energy minimization approach to study several possible binding modes of steroid diamines to three different double-stranded DNA sequences.

Steroid-Binding Proteins

Absent from this list are modeling and simulation studies of steroid-protein binding, an especially notable absence in light of the popularity of ligand-protein binding in other areas of drug design. Probably the major reason for this is a lack of molecular structures of steroid-binding proteins. Of primary interest would be the hormone-binding domain of steroid receptors. Unfortunately, although a substantial amount is known of the sequence, biochemistry and action of these proteins [73], their substantial posttranslational modification diminishes the advantages provided by the methods of cloning and overexpression, a primary means of obtaining the large quantities of protein required for structure determination. One study used computational methods to develop a model of one hormone-binding domain based on a proposed similarity to proteins whose structures are known [74]. The DNA-binding domain of the glucocorticoid receptor, highly conserved across the family of nuclear transcription factors, has recently been determined using NMR [75]. However, this portion of the receptor is of much less interest in drug design than the hormone-binding domain. Often examination of the binding and function of one protein can help in understanding a related protein. To date, the X-ray crystallographically derived structures of 5 steroid-binding proteins have been determined: uteroglobin, a progesterone-binding protein [76]; hydroxysteroid dehydrogenase [77]; cholesterol oxidase [78], and two antibodies that bind steroid-like molecules [P. Jeffrey, pers. communication].

Conclusions

CADD constitutes the application of a diverse group of methods for the elucidation of complicated biochemical phenomena. Although many of the methods are still experimental, there have already been documented successes and the future is promising. Computational methods are progressively becoming more refined, as is chemists' capability for applying them. The primary impediment of many of the computational approaches is lack of computing power, a weakness that is rapidly diminishing due to the dramatic increase in speed and capacity and parallel decrease in price of computing platforms.

In the limited space of this paper, it was impossible to provide anything but an enumeration and brief introduction to the major methods of computational chemistry that have been applied to drug design problems. The references provided here for each of the methods constitute more thorough introductions and review.

Computational study of steroids is a well-established field having been conducted now for several decades on a number of classes of steroids and for several different physical properties and biological activities.

References

1   Cohen NC, Blaney JM, Humblet C, Gund P, Berry DC: Molecular Modeling Software and Methods for Medicinal Chemistry. J Med Chem 1990;33:883–894.
2   Dearing A: Computer-aided molecular modelling: Research study or research tool? J Comput Aided Mol Des 1988;2:179–189.
3   Boyd DB: Aspects of molecular modeling; in Lipkowitz KB, Boyd DB (eds): Reviews in Computational Chemistry. New York, VCH, 1990, vol 1, pp 321–354.
4   Boyd DB, Lipkowitz KB: Molecular mechanics: The method and its underlying philosophy. J Chem Education 1982;59:269–274.
5   Burkert U, Allinger NL: Molecular Mechanics. ACS Monograph 177. Washington, American Chemical Society, 1982.
6   Allinger NL, Li F, Yan L, Tai JC: Molecular mechanics (MM3) calculations on conjugated hydrocarbons. J Comput Chem 1990;11:868–895.
7   Dinur U, Hagher AT: New approaches to empirical force fields; in Lipkowitz KB, Boyd DB (eds): Reviews in Computational Chemistry. New York, VCH, 1990, vol 2, pp 99–164.
8   Bowen JP, Allinger NL: Molecular mechanics: The art and science of parameterization; in Lipkowitz KB, Boyd DB (eds): Reviews in Computational Chemistry. New York, VCH, 1990, vol 2, pp 81–98.
9   Brunger AT, Kuriyan J, Karplus M: Crystallographic R factor refinement by molecular dynamics. Science 1987;235:458–460.

10   Struthers RS, Tanaka G, Koerber SC, Solmajer T, Baniak EL, Gierasch LM, Vale W, Rivier J, Hagler AT: Design of biologically active, conformationally constrained GnRH antagonists. Proteins 1990;8:295–304.

11   McCammon JA, Harvey SC: Dynamics of Proteins and Nucleic Acids. New York, Cambridge University Press, 1989.

12   Stewart JJP: Semiempirical molecular orbital methods; in Lipkowitz KB, Boyd DB (eds): Reviews in Computational Chemistry. New York, VCH, 1990, vol 1, pp 45–82.

13   Zerner MC: Semiempirical molecular orbital methods; in Lipkowitz KB, Boyd DB (eds): Reviews in Computational Chemistry. New York, VCH, 1990, vol 2, pp 313–366.

14   Howard A, Kollman PA: An analysis of current methodologies for conformational searching of complex molecules. J Med Chem 1988;31:1669–1675.

15   Saunders M, Houk KN, Wu Y, Still WC, Lipton M, Chang G, Guida WC: Conformations of cycloheptadecane. A comparison of methods for conformational searching. J Am Chem Soc 1990;112:1419–1427.

16   Leach AR: A survey of methods for searching the conformational space of small and medium-sized molecules; in Lipkowitz KB, Boyd DB (eds): Reviews in Computational Chemistry. New York, VCH, 1990, vol 2, pp 1–56.

17   Rushinko A, III, Sheridan RP, Nilakantan R, Karaki KS, Bauman N, Venkatarachavan R: Using CONCORD to construct a large database of the three-dimensional coordinates from connection tables. J Chem Inf Comput Sci 1989;29:251–255.

18   Martin YC: 3D database searching in drug design. J Med Chem 1992;35:2145–2154.

19   Martin YC, Bures MG, Willet P: Searching databases of three-dimensional structures; in Lipkowitz KB, Boyd DB (eds): Reviews in Computational Chemistry. New York, VCH, 1990, vol 1, pp 214–264.

20   Boyd DB: Successes of computer-assisted molecular design; in Lipkowitz KB, Boyd DB (eds): Reviews in Computational Chemistry. New York, VCH, 1990, vol 1, pp 355–372.

21   Martin YC: Quantitative Drug Design: A Critical Introduction. New York, Dekker, 1978.

22   Martin YC: Modern Drug Research. New York, Dekker, 1989.

23   Martin YC: A practitioner's perspective of the role of quantitative structure-activity analysis in medicinal chemistry. J Med Chem 1981;24:229–237.

24   Plummer EL: The application of quantitative design strategies in pesticide discovery; in Lipkowitz KB, Boyd DB (eds): Reviews in Computational Chemistry. New York, VCH, 1990, vol 1, pp 119–168.

25   Marshall GR, Motoc I: Approaches to the conformation of the drug bound to the receptor; in Burgen ASV, Roberts GCK, Tute MS (eds): Molecular Graphics and Drug Design. Topics in Molecular Pharmacology. Amsterdam, Elsevier, 1986, vol 3, p 115.

26   Cramer RD, III, Patterson DE, Bunce JD: Comparative molecular field analysis (CoMFA). 1. Effect of shape on binding of steroids to carrier proteins. J Am Chem Soc 1998;110:5959–5967.

27   Troyer JM, Cohen FE: Simplified models for understanding and predicting protein structure; in Lipkowitz KB, Boyd DB (eds): Reviews in Computational Chemistry. New York, VCH, 1990, vol 2, pp 57–74.

28   Dill KA: Dominant forces in protein folding. Biochemistry 1990;29:7133–7155.

29   Fasman GD (ed): Prediction of Protein Structure and the Principles of Protein Conformation. New York, Plenum, 1989.

30   Goodford PJ: A computational procedure for determining energetically favorable binding sites on biologically important molecules. J Med Chem 1985;28:849–857.

31   Kuntz ID: Structure-based strategies for drug design and discovery. Science 1992;257:1078–1082.

32   Lybrand TP: Computer simulation of biomolecular systems using molecular dynamics and free energy perturbation methods; in Lipkowitz KB, Boyd DB (eds): Reviews in Computational Chemistry. New York, VCH, 1990, vol 1, pp 295–320.

33   van Gunsteren WF, Weiner PK (eds): Computer Simulation of Biomolecular Systems. Leiden, Escom, 1989.

34   Hansch C, Klein TE: Molecular graphics and QSAR in the study of enzyme-ligand interactions. On the definition of bioreceptors. Acc Chem Res 1986;19:392.

35   Hansch C: On the state of QSAR. Drug Inf J 1984;18:115–122.

---

36   Boyd DB: The computational chemistry literature; in Lipkowitz KB, Boyd DB (eds): Reviews in Computational Chemistry. New York, VCH, 1990, vol 2, pp 461–477.

37   Lipkowitz KB, Boyd DB (eds): Reviews in Computational Chemistry. New York, VCH, 1990, vol 1.

38   Lipkowitz KB, Boyd DB (eds): Reviews in Computational Chemistry. New York, VCH, 1990, vol 2.

39   Clark T: A Handbook of Computational Chemistry. New York, Wiley, 1985.

40   Hirst DM: A Computational Approach to Chemistry. Boston, Blackwell, 1990.

41   Ambos MM, Gelin BR, Richon AB: The Computational Chemistry Yellow Pages. St. Louis, Custom Research and Consulting and Molecular Solutions, Inc., 1992.

42   Quantum Chemistry Program Exchange. Creative Arts Building 181, Indiana University, Bloomington, IN 47405 (USA), Tel. (812)855-4784/FAX: (812) 855-5539.

43   Boyd DB: Appendix: Compendium of software for molecular modeling; in Lipkowitz KB, Boyd DB (eds): Reviews in Computational Chemistry. New York, VCH, 1990, vol 1, pp 383–392.

44   Boyd DB: Appendix: Compendium of software for molecular modeling; in Lipkowitz KB, Boyd DB (eds): Reviews in Computational Chemistry. New York, VCH, 1990, vol 2, pp 481–498.

45   Wolff ME, et al: Correlation of glucocorticoid and progestational activity with steric electronic and hydrophobic parameters. J Steroid Biochem 1975;6:211–214.

46   Schmit JP, Rousseau GG: Structure and conformation of glucocorticoids; in Wolff ME (ed): Glucocorticoid Hormone Action. New York, Springer, 1979, p 79–95.

47   Wolff ME: In Wolff ME (ed): Bruger's Medicinal Chemistry, ed 4. New York, Wiley, 1980, part III, p 1273.

48   Schmit JP, Rousseau GG: Structure-activity relationships for glucocorticoids. III. Structural and conformational study of the rings and side-chain of steroids which bind to the glucocorticoid receptor. J Steroid Biochem 1978;9:909–920.

49   Schmit JP, Rousseau GG: Structure-activity relationships for glucocorticoids. IV. Effects of substituents on the overall shape of steroids which bind to the glucocorticoid receptor. J Steroid Biochem 1978;9:921–927.

50   Kollman PA, Giannini DD, Duax WL, Rothenberg S, Wolff ME: Quantitation of long-range effects in steroids by molecular orbital calculations. J Am Chem Soc 1973;95:2869.

51   Wolff ME: Quantitative Structure-Activity Relationships. Budapest, Akademiai Kiado, 1973, p 31.

52   Bohl M, Sussmilch R: Calculations on molecular structure and electrostatic potentials of cardiotonic steroids. Eur J Med Chem Chim Ther 1986;21:193–198.

53   Pasa-Tolic LJ, Klasinc L, Spiegl H, Knop JV, McGlynn SP: Ab initio calculations on 5α-androstane. Int J Quant Chem 1992;41:815–827.

54   Bohl M: Molecular mechanics investigation on side-chain conformations of a 17α-ethyl-17beta-hydroxy steroid with regard to receptor binding. Z Naturforsch, C.: Biosci 1987;42:221–224.

55   Li P, Brueggemeier RW: 7-Substituted steroidal aromatase inhibitors: Structure-activity relationships and molecular modeling. J Enzyme Inhib 1990;4:113–120.

56   White P, Breslow R: Molecular mechanics calculations on template-directed steroid chlorinations: Are transition states rigidified by the geometric trajectory requirements for effective energy transfer? J Am Chem Soc 1990;112:6842–6847.

57   Dunn WJ, III, Koehler MG, Grigoras S: The role of solvent-accessible surface area in determining partition coefficients. Med Chem 1987;30:1121–1126.

58   Ormerod A, Willett P, Bawden D: Comparison of fragment weighting schemes for substructural analysis. Quant Struct Act Relat 1989;8:115–129.

59   Pepperrell CA, Willett P: Techniques for the calculation of three-dimensional structural similarity using inter-atomic distances. J Comput Aided Mol Des 1991;5:455–474.

60   Rum G, Herndon WC: Molecular similarity concepts. 5. Analysis of steroid-protein binding constants. J Am Chem Soc 1991;113:9055–9060.

61   Bodor N, Harget AJ, Phillips EW: Structure-activity relationships in the antiinflammatory steroids: A pattern-recognition approach. J Med Chem 1983;26:318–328.

62   Stouch TR, Jurs PC: Pattern recognition studies of the structure-activity relationships of antiinflammatory steroids. J Med Chem 1986;29:2125–2136.

63   Stouch TR: Structure-activity relationships using multivariate analysis techniques: Application to topical corticosteroids; in Maibach HI, Surber C (eds): Topical Corticosteroids. Basel, Karger, 1992, pp 93–127.

64   Ebert E, Eckhardt E, Jakel K, Moser P, Sozzi D, Vogel C: Quantitative structure activity relationships of fungicidally active triazoles: Analogs and stereoisomers of propiconazole and etaconazole. Z Naturforsch, C.: Biosci 1989;44:85–96.

65   Zeelen FJ: QSAR of steroids. Quant Struct Act Relat 1986;5:131–137.

66   Simon Z, Bohl M: Structure-activity relations in gestagenic steroids by the MTD method. The case of hard molecules and soft receptors. Quant Struct Act Relat 1992;11:23–28.

67   Bohl M, Simon Z, Lochmann JR: Theoretical investigations on the role of steroid-skeleton C4–C5 unsaturation in competitive aromatase inhibition. Z Naturforsch, C.: Biosci 1989;44:217–225.

68   Kellogg GE, Semus SF, Abraham DJ: HINT: A new method of empirical hydrophobic field calculation for CoMFA. J Comput Aided Mol Des 1991;5:545–552.

69   Norinder U: Experimental design based 3-D QSAR analysis of steroid-protein interactions: Application to human CBG complexes. J Comput Aided Mol Des 1990;4:381–389.

70   Norinder U: 3-D QSAR analysis of steroid/protein interactions: The use of difference maps. J Comput Aided Mol Des 1991;5:419–426.

71   Laughton CA, Neidle S: Inhibitors of the P450 enzymes aromatase and lyase. Crystallographic and molecular modeling studies suggest structural features of pyridylacetic acid derivatives responsible for differences in enzyme inhibitory activity. J Med Chem 1990;33:3055–3060.

72   Hui X, Gresh N, Pullman B: Modeling basic features of specificity in the binding of a dicationic steroid diamine to double-stranded oligonucleotides. Nucleic Acids Res 1989;17:4177–4187.

73   Agarwal MK: Steroid receptor structure and antihormone drug design. Biochem Pharmacol 1992; 43:2299–2306.

74   Lemesle-Varloot L, Ojasso T, Momon JP, Raynaud JP: A model for the determination of the 3D-spatial distribution of the hormone-binding domain of receptors that bind 3-keto-4-ene steroids. J Steroid Biochem Mol Biol 1992;41:369–388.

75   Hard T, Kellenbach E, Boelens R, Maler BA, Dahlman K, Feedman LP, Carlstedt-Duke J, Yamamoto KR, Gustafsson J, Kaptein R: Solution structure of the glucocorticoid receptor DNA-binding domain. Science 1990;249:157–160.

76   Bally R, Delettre J: Structure and refinement of the oxidized P2 = 1 = form of uteroglobin at 1.64 Ångström resolution. J Mol Biol 1989;206:153–170.

77   Ghosh D, Weeks CM, Grochulski P, Duax WL, Erman M, Rimsay RL, Orr JC: Three-dimensional structure of holo 3α,20β-hydroxysteroid dehydrogenase: A member of a short-*chain dehydrogenase family. Proc Natl Acad Sci USA 1991;88:10064–10068.

78   Vrielink A, Lloyd AF, Blow DM: Crystal structure of cholesterol oxidase from Brevibacterium sterolicum refined at 1.8 Ångströms resolution. J Mol Biol 1991;219:533.

Terry R. Stouch, PhD, Room H3812, Bristol-Myers Squibb Pharmaceutical Research Institute, PO Box 4000, Princeton, NJ 08543-4000 (USA)

Korting HC, Maibach HI (eds): Topical Glucocorticoids with Increased Benefit/Risk Ratio.
Curr Probl Dermatol. Basel, Karger, 1993, vol 21, pp 45–60

....

Percutaneous Absorption of Topical Corticosteroids

Ronald C. Wester, Howard I. Maibach

Department of Dermatology, University of California, San Francisco, Calif., USA

Studies that examine the pharmacokinetics of topical drugs at their site of action in the skin have been difficult to perform and are therefore limited in number. In the early years of topical drug pharmacokinetic research, investigators had to rely on the measurement of less direct indicators of drug throughput such as blood levels and urinary excretion. Today, advances in theory are impelling pharmacokinetic research in new directions, including the measurement of drug availability in tissue compartments within the skin. This research will lead to greater precision in pharmacokinetic measurement and greater relevance of these measurements to the therapeutic efficacy of topical corticosteroids in cutaneous disease states.

Investigations of the pharmacokinetic properties of topically applied chemicals have shown that their concentrations in tape-stripped stratum corneum may be well correlated with cumulative urinary excretion, blood levels and other measurements of systemic drug absorption. However, research that examines the pharmacokinetics of topical drugs at their site of action in the skin has been difficult to perform and is therefore limited. Detailed knowledge of what happens to a topical agent in the tissue compartment where it has its therapeutic activity should greatly facilitate our ability to develop a method to test topical corticosteroid bioequivalence.

This paper not only summarizes recent advances in our knowledge of the dermatopharmacokinetics of topical corticosteroids, but also identifies the gaps that exist in this knowledge.

Individual Variation

Measurements of urinary excretion of radiolabeled, topically applied corticosteroids in subjects with normal skin have shown marked interindividual variations in absorption kinetics. In one study performed more than 20 years ago [1], we measured 5-day urinary excretion of ^{14}C-hydrocortisone, which was applied to the ventral forearm in a dose of 4 μg/cm^2, in 18 normal volunteers. In 4 of the subjects, total urinary drug excretion was about one fourth the median value; in a fifth subject, this measurement indicated absorption of 3 times the median amount of drug.

In another experiment [unpubl. data], Patrick Noonan measured blood levels of nitroglycerin after topical application of 2 doses: 20 and 40 μg/cm^2. although there was great variation among subjects in the amount of nitroglycerin absorbed transdermally, each subject was highly consistent in the percent of absorbed dose for each of the 2 dose levels. These findings suggest that investigators of topical corticosteroid pharmacokinetics may benefit from this within-subject consistency by designing their experiments so that each subject serves as his or her own control. Furthermore, it is likely that minimal absorbers will present a greater therapeutic challenge and hyperabsorbers are presumably more at risk for adverse effects.

Rougier et al. [2] documented a high correlation between transepidermal water loss in vivo in man and percutaneous penetration of 4 chemicals of differing physicochemical properties. Should this correlation hold up in studies with a broader range of chemicals, it should be possible at the bedside or in the laboratory to predict the relative permeability of a given individual. The robust nature of such a prediction is obvious.

Repeated Topical Drug Applications

Of course we do not treat our patients with a single application of a topical corticosteroid, and hence should not assume that weeks or years of corticoid application do not alter the permeability of the skin. In a rhesus monkey model, Wester et al. [3] showed that prolonged application of hydrocortisone altered the barrier function of the stratum corneum, resulting in enhanced drug penetration. In this rhesus monkey model, a single dose of ^{14}C-labeled hydrocortisone was applied at baseline and then once again after long-term administration of nonradioactive hydrocortisone. Percutaneous absorption of labeled hydrocortisone was markedly increased after 8 days of hydrocortisone administration, and the effect was consistent between ointment and acetone vehicles.

Table 1. Expected and observed hydrocortisone absorption in man

Treatment No.	Dosing sequence	Hydrocortisone absorbed, $\mu g/cm^2$	
		expected	observed
1	13.3 $\mu g/cm^2$ × 1	–	0.056
2	40.0 $\mu g/cm^2$ × 1	0.168[a]	0.140
3	13.33 $\mu g/cm^2$ × 3 (no wash)	0.168[a]	0.372
4	13.33 $\mu g/cm^2$ × 3 (wash)	0.168[a]	0.472

The values of hydrocortisone absorbed are average amount absorbed from 6 volunteers.
[a] Expected values are 0.056 $\mu g/cm^2$ × 3 = 0.168 $\mu g/cm^2$.

However, our replication of these observations in human subjects provides a cautionary example about extrapolation of animal data to humans. In these studies, conducted by Bucks et al. [4, 5], the experimental design in the rhesus monkeys was duplicated, with minor but perhaps important modification, in 5 healthy human subjects. A major difference in design resided in the utilization of a nonocclusive protective device in the man minimizing rub-off, and the lack thereof in the rhesus. Eight days of daily hydrocortisone application failed to alter percutaneous absorption of ^{14}C-labeled hydrocortisone.

An investigation was designed to determine if multiple-dose therapy (dosing the same site 3 times in the same day) would increase drug bioavailability in human skin [6]. Percutaneous absorption of hydrocortisone was measured in 6 healthy adult men from whom informed consent had been obtained. The study compared treatment with a single topical dose to treatment with multiple doses (1 vs. 3 applications) in the same day. ^{14}C-labeled hydrocortisone in acetone was applied to 2.5 cm^2 of ventral forearm skin and protected with a nonocclusive polypropylene chamber. The amount of ^{14}C measured in urine collected over 7 days was used to determine hydrocortisone absorption. The treatments, performed 2–3 weeks apart, each utilized adjacent sites on the same individuals (table 1). A single dose of hydrocortisone (13.33 $\mu g/cm^2$) delivered a mass of 0.056 $\mu g/cm^2$. Three serial doses of 13.33 $\mu g/cm^2$ (total 40 $\mu g/cm^2$) were also expected to deliver 0.168 $\mu g/cm^2$ with or without soap and water washing between doses, but the observed amount of hydrocortisone delivered significantly exceeded the expected mass absorbed. This indicates that multiple-dosing treatments resulted in a significant increase in bioavailability – when dosing was the same day (table 1). It is postulated that increased acetone vehicle application and skin washing dissolved and mobilized previously dosed hydrocortisone and increased bioavailability. This common dosing situation in clinical practice deserves further experimentation with different vehicles and chemicals.

Factors That Affect Corticosteroid Penetration

In clinical situations, manipulations such as occlusion, duration and frequency of daily dosing, and the concentration of active drug may at least theoretically alter the amount of drug that enters the skin. Experimental evidence suggests that we can usually but not always count on these manipulations to have their desired effects.

Occlusion

A dogma of topical corticosteroid therapy is that occlusion increases the efficacy of any given formulation. Occlusion has been shown to enhance both the pharmacodynamic effect of corticosteroids (in the vasoconstrictor assay [7]) and total drug throughput, measured by urinary drug excretion [8]. In the latter experiment, total urinary hydrocortisone excretion was increased 10-fold by occluding the skin for 96 h after the corticosteroid was applied. In a subsequent experiment, we applied labeled hydrocortisone to the skin under 24-hour occlusion, a procedure that is more like real-life clinical applications. In that study, occlusion had no effect on the amount of hydrocortisone absorbed [9]. One must conclude, while the ability of occlusion to enhance drug efficacy and pharmacodynamics is undeniable, this enhancement may not necessarily be achieved by increasing skin penetration of the active agent – at least in short-term (24 h) application. The dynamic effect may be related to differential deposition in blood vessel compartments not assayable with current methodology.

Duration of Topical Application

Typically we instruct our patients to apply corticosteroids to the skin for many hours, several times daily. Research is also challenging these dogmas of topical therapy. For some topical agents, a brief application may be sufficient to produce complete residence within the tissue compartment in which the agent is active. In a study in which betamethasone dipropionate was applied to the skin under occlusion and washed off after 20 min, clinical efficacy was unimpaired. Incidentally, in this study the brief application of drug did not result in skin blanching, unlike the longer application. These observations suggest that, whatever methods are adopted to make bioequivalence, comparison of topical corticosteroids will have to address measurements that are relevant to these agents' clinical effects.

Manufacturers of oral drugs have realized that patients' compliance with therapy is increased by offering them once-daily dosage. Dermatologic tradition and drug packaging still often uphold the practice of applying topical corticosteroids several times daily. However, in a recent clinical trial, once-daily application of halcinonide was often as efficacious as multiple daily doses. Previously, we had shown that total absorption and excretion of radiolabeled hydrocortisone in rhesus monkeys was not substantially increased when a 13.3-$\mu g/cm^2$ dose of the corticoid was applied 3 times a day instead of once a day [10]. It is interesting that, in this model, total absorption was markedly increased when the entire daily dose of $40\ \mu g/cm^2$ was applied at once rather than at 3 separate times.

Concentration of the Active Compound

In an early experiment, we compared percutaneous absorption of increasing concentrations of ^{14}C-hydrocortisone in rhesus monkeys and human subjects [11]. In the monkeys, 5 different concentrations of active drug, ranging from 40 to $4,000\ \mu g/cm^2$, dissolved in acetone, were applied to the skin. In human subjects, concentrations of 4 and $40\ \mu g/cm^2$ were applied. In both species, total absorption increased as a function of increasing drug concentrations; however, the efficiency of absorption decreased. In the human subjects, the 10-fold increase in applied drug concentration resulted in 4-fold greater drug absorption, but a decrease in the efficiency of absorption from 1.6 to 0.6%. Similar studies have not been published for other topical corticosteroids or other vehicle formulations, though Stoughton and Wullich [12] have shown that different concentrations of active drug in several commercially available corticosteroids do not produce different degrees of skin blanching in the vasoconstrictor assay.

These dose-response relationships, both in terms of pharmacokinetics and clinical response, require further detailed exploration. Increasingly higher concentrations were commercialized on intuitive grounds, e.g. triamcinolone acetonide 0.025, 0.1, 0.5%. Furthermore, early studies with the small-plaque psoriasis assay supported this assumption. Yet, the opposite observations in some of the recent Stoughton and Wullich experiments [12] call for a reexamination of dogma.

Regional Variation

Feldmann and Maibach [13] were the first scientists to explore the potential for regional variation in percutaneous absorption. The first absorption studies were done with the ventral forearm, because this site is convenient to use. However, skin exposure to chemicals exists over the whole body. They first showed regional variation with the absorption of hydrocortisone. The scrotum was the highest-absorbing skin site (the first recognized occupational disease was scrotal cancer in chimney sweeps – scrotal skin absorption is the key). Skin absorption

Table 2. Penetration indices for 5 anatomical sites assessed using hydrocortisone skin penetration data in man

Site	Penetration index based on hydrocortisone
Genitals (scrotum)	40
Arms (forearm)	1
Legs	0.5
Trunk	2.5
Head	5

From Feldmann and Maibach [13] and Guy and Maibach [14].

was lowest for the foot area and highest around the head and face. Regional variation in man was later confirmed with other chemicals. Guy and Maibach [14] took the hydrocortisone data and constructed penetration indices for 5 anatomical sites (table 2). These indices should be used with their total surface areas when considering systemic availability relative to body exposure sites.

Most of what we know about topical corticosteroid penetration relates to the human forearm. Investigators have justifiably avoided introducing another source of variability into their experiments of percutaneous penetration by testing different anatomical regions. In the above experiment we showed that absorption was increased as much as 13-fold in the angle of the jaw and 40-fold on the scrotum, compared with the ventral forearm.

Unfortunately, even the forearm is not as uniform a test site as one would like. We recently produced data showing a gradient in absorption from the top to the bottom of the forearm. This gradient should be built in to any experimental design that uses the forearm for tape-stripping or other assays of topical drug penetration.

Effect of the Vehicle

Vehicles and other formulation factors can affect not only the absorption of a topical drug but also its clinical effect. In an in vivo hairless rat model, Rougier et al. [2] showed that simple modifications in the vehicle could result in 50-fold differences in penetration of benzoic acid. In this study, drug concentrations in tape-stripped stratum corneum were linearly correlated with 4-day drug excretion, a finding that has obvious implications for investigators wishing to develop

Table 3. Penetration of hydrocortisone through modified human skin in vivo

Treatment	Penetration ratio
None	1
Strip (cellophane tape)	4
Occlude (Saran® plastic wrap)	10
Cantharidin blister	16
Strip + occlude	20

models to measure vehicle effects. In human studies with single vehicles (mineral oil, dimethylformamide, dimethylacetonide, propylene glycol and dimethyl sulfoxide), the variation approximated 4-fold.

Diseased Skin

Percutaneous absorption of dermatological drugs is usually determined on human volunteers or animals with intact skin. An 'estimate' of absorption for diseased skin is then determined by inflicting some trauma to the skin as a model system. This extends from the assumption that diseased skin is damaged skin. The assumption then follows that percutaneous absorption through diseased/damaged skin is enhanced, and that the skin's ability to protect against intrusion by chemicals is impaired.

Most models for diseased skin extend from the original publications of Feldmann and Maibach [8, 9] and Wester and Maibach [15]. Various physical procedures are used to disrupt the so-called 'barrier' to percutaneous absorption. Skin stripping is the application of a strip of cellophane tape to skin which removes a layer of stratum corneum when the tape is pulled off the skin. When this is repeated 10–20 times, a 'glistening layer' is reached. Cantharidin solution topically applied to skin induces a blister (which will heal without leaving a scar). Occlusion is defined as the physical covering of skin after a chemical is applied to the skin surface. Occlusion prevents loss of compound and forces changes in humidity and temperature. Occlusion in the laboratory is accomplished by use of a covering of plastic wrap, which represents the most extreme occlusive condition.

Table 3 gives the penetration ratios of hydrocortisone when human skin in vivo is modified by stripping, occlusion and blistering. These physical procedures

Table 4. Percutaneous absorption in psoriasis

Drug/chemical	Result	Reference
Hydrocortisone	no difference	Wester et al. [16]
Anthralin	no difference	Wester et al. [17]
Anthralin	increase	Wang et al. [18]
Triamcinolone	increase	Schaefer et al. [19]
		Schalla et al. [20]
5-Fluorouracil	increase	Erlanger et al. [21]
Nandrolone	no difference	Foreman et al. [22]
Salts	increase	Shani [23]
Water loss	increase	Grice et al. [24]

increase the penetration ratio of hydrocortisone beyond that of unmodified skin. However, even with these destructive methods, removing most of the stratum corneum does not remove the skin's ability to protect against intrusion by chemicals.

Psoriasis is a common chronic squamous dermatosis, characterized clinically by the presence of rounded, circumscribed, erythematous, dry scaling patches covered by grayish white or silvery white, umbilicated lamellar scales. Table 4 lists the studies on percutaneous absorption in psoriasis for several drugs and other chemicals [16–24]. The results list whether there was a difference in percutaneous absorption between normal human skin and psoriatic skin. There is disagreement, and these differences are probably due to variables within the study designs. Besides differences in drug or chemical studies, there were differences in skin pretreatment and vehicles [16–24].

Wester et al. [16] determined the percutaneous absorption of the corticoid hydrocortisone formulated as a 0.5% cream (Cort-Dome). Percutaneous absorption as measured by urinary excretion (with parenteral control) for normal volunteers was 2.4 ± (SD) 1.2% of the topically applied dose for a 24-hour skin application time. Patients hospitalized for psoriasis were treated in the same manner as normal volunteers. Note that there was no pretreatment of the psoriatic plaques before the hydrocortisone was applied. Percutaneous absorption in psoriatic patients was 2.3 ± 1.4%, a value not statistically different from normal volunteers.

Foreman et al. [22] studied the in vitro diffusion of the corticoid nandrolone through human cadaver skin. The skin absorption through psoriatic skin was the same as normal skin, which in turn was not much different if skin was occluded or stripped.

Table 5. Percutaneous absorption of hydrocortisone with various skin conditions

Species	Skin condition	Percent dose absorbed	Reference
Human	normal	2.3 ± 1.4	Wester et al. [16]
	psoriatic	2.4 ± 1.2	
Human	normal	0.5 ± 0.2	Feldmann and Maibach [8, 9]
	tape-stripped	0.9 ± 0.5	
	occluded	5.3 ± 2.6	
	strip + occlude	14.9 ± 6.5	
Human	normal	1.1 ± 0.3	Bucks et al. [25]
	delipidized	1.1 ± 0.5	
Human	normal	4.4 ± 1.7	Bucks et al. [26]
	occluded	4.0 ± 2.4	
	multiple dose	3.1 ± 1.0	
Rhesus monkey	uninvolved	2.6 ± 0.1	Bronaugh et al. [27]
	eczematous dermatitis	5.5 ± 0.7	
Rhesus monkey	normal	0.5 ± 0.04	Wester et al. [28]
	multiple dose	1.9 ± 0.4	

Values are mean ± SD.

Table 5 summarizes the data for percutaneous absorption of hydrocortisone where some skin condition, either mechanical (tape strip, occlude), biological (de-lipidize, multiple dose) or diseased (psoriatic, eczematous), was directly compared to normal control skin [25–28]. What is of most interest is that all percent doses absorbed over a 24-hour skin application time are 5% or less of the applied dose (except where skin was tape-stripped and occluded). The ability of skin to maintain barrier properties relative to hydrocortisone for the variety of treatments is impressive.

Table 6 summarizes the changes in serum hydrocortisone following topical hydrocortisone application for dermatitis in adults and children [29, 30]. The methodology was to first suppress adrenal production of endogenous hydrocortisone with dexamethasone injections. Then hydrocortisone was topically administered to dermatitis patients. Adult atopic dermatitis patients were classified as: (1) widespread and high-grade erythema; (2) widespread and low-grade, and (3) complete remission. Postapplication rise in serum hydrocortisone was greater

Table 6. Serum hydrocortisone following topical hydrocortisone application for dermatitis

| Dermatitis | Mean hydrocortisone levels, nM | | | | |
| | children | | | adults | |
	<18 months	>18 months	all	median	range
Severe	807±718	268±204	537±589	314	18–711
Moderate	257±218	135±81	193±175	114	29–680
Mild	132±56	78±54	107±54	10	0–65

Values given for children are mean ± SD. [Adapted from ref. 29 and 30.]

for acute dermatitis patients (groups 1 and 2) than for patients in complete remission (group 3). The children were patients with atopic or seborrheic dermatitis. There was a higher rise of serum hydrocortisone in children with severe dermatitis than in children with moderate dermatitis. Children with mild dermatitis had lower serum hydrocortisone than children with moderate dermatitis. Serum hydrocortisone in children under 18 months with severe dermatitis was significantly greater than in children over 18 months with mild dermatitis. Separate studies were done with children and with adults, so direct statistical comparison between children and adults cannot be done.

The data in table 5 suggest that hydrocortisone percutaneous absorption is relatively immune to changes in skin condition. Data from table 6 suggest the opposite, especially for severe dermatitis. A variable in the two data presentations is skin surface area and this may explain the results. In the experimentally controlled studies (table 5) surface area is constant. In treating skin disease the more severe indication may mean a larger area of involvement (larger surface area).

Among the numerous animal models for percutaneous absorption, there are a multiplicity of skin diseases that animals can acquire and considerable treatments which can be utilized. The percutaneous absorption of hydrocortisone and benzoic acid was compared between normal hairless guinea pig skin and damaged skin [31]. Another example of an animal model is the creation of epidermal hyperproliferation in normal hairless mice and rats due to essential fatty acid deficiency (EFAD). The skin appears drier and with more dandruff-like scaliness. Percutaneous absorption of hydrocortisone was 31.3% in control mice and 59.3% in EFAD mice [32]. Difference in water loss from skin increased at day 20 for EFAD rats [33]. In all of these model systems the key will be in determining the relevance of the animal and the skin treatment/disease to that of man.

The assumption proposed in the introduction to this paper was that percutaneous absorption through diseased/damaged skin is enhanced, and that the skin's ability to protect against intrusion by chemicals is impaired. The picture of skin flood gates opening and chemicals pouring in is certainly not warranted (except perhaps in severe burn or erythroderma cases). The data suggest that diseased skin can retain barrier properties, and that differences will exist for different drugs and for different disease conditions. However, even for a compound such as hydrocortisone where skin absorption is low for diseased and damaged skin, enhanced absorption will occur in severe conditions (as Turpeinen reported for severe dermatitis in younger children). For more potent corticosteroids the risk of systemic side effects such as adrenal suppression remains real.

In vitro percutaneous absorption and throughput of hydrocortisone and 3 nonsteroidal compounds was increased in a guinea pig model by including an irritant dermatitis with sodium lauryl sulfate [34]. In this experiment, cumulative absorption was enhanced by dermatitis to a greater degree than drug concentration in the skin, and enhancement of absorption was greater for hydrophilic than for lipophilic compounds. Experimental studies in human subjects and animal models show that the effect of skin damage on barrier function depends on factors including the mechanism of skin damage, the physicochemical characteristics of the test substance, and other aspects of experimental design. However, the general tendency is for skin disease or injury to increase percutaneous absorption [35].

Spontaneously occurring cutaneous disease states in humans may vary in their effect on percutaneous drug absorption. Psoriatic skin is less permeable than healthy skin, a finding which may explain why psoriasis is often so difficult to treat with topical agents [36].

Bioavailability and Bioequivalence

Corticosteroids when applied to the skin exert a specific pharmacological response that is evident as skin blanching. This pharmacodynamic response depends on the potency of the steroid, the drug release properties of the formulation and the bioavailability/pharmacokinetic behavior of the drug in the skin. The skin blanching assay is a qualitative assessment, subject to all of the parameters involved. Bioavailability refers to the rate and extent of drug appearance at the target site (skin) or the systemic circulation. The actual concentration of drug is measured at the target site or in the systemic circulation to give a quantitative amount. Comparing two dosage forms in the same test assay will determine bioequivalence between the two dosage forms. The skin blanching test can give a qualitative equivalence but the dosage forms may not be bioequivalent because the bioavailability/actual drug concentrations in the skin may be different. Relationships between skin blanching, vehicle release rates and skin drug content need to be established to determine actual bioavailability and bioequivalence [37, 38].

Relevance of Animal Models and in vitro Test Systems

Animal Models of Percutaneous Absorption

In vivo animal models for percutaneous absorption have included many species: the albino rabbit, miniature swine, rhesus monkey, spider monkey, guinea pig, and various rat and mouse species among others. These animal models vary in efficiency of percutaneous absorption and therefore in their relevance to humans. Proposed explanations for this variance include differences in skin thickness, in the lipid content of skin and in test methods that have been used to measure penetration, which may in part be beyond the investigator's control [39]. Bartek et al. [40] showed that, in in vivo studies attempting to measure the potential for dermal toxicity, the miniature swine model provides a close approximation of a human skin permeability, while rat and rabbit models had considerably greater skin permeability than either swine or the human subjects. Skin permeability in monkey species also resembles that of humans fairly closely. These observations do not imply that investigators should not perform studies of percutaneous absorption in the less expensive and more accessible rabbit and rat laboratory models, only that the methods used in these studies should be fully described and the results extrapolated to humans with care.

In vitro-in vivo Correlations

In vitro models of percutaneous absorption allow investigators to examine percutaneous absorption more directly than living systems by measuring absorption directly below the skin membrane, a design which removes systemic pharmacokinetics as a source of possible confounding. Typically a passive diffusion system such as the static Franz diffusion cell is used with skin membrane preparations from humans or animals. Comparative studies have shown that percutaneous absorption in in vivo and in vitro models is usually parallel across species; that is, the in vitro penetration characteristics of human skin resemble pig and monkey skin more closely than rat, rabbit or guinea pig skin [41].

In humans, published reports of direct comparisons between in vivo and in vitro absorption include only about 10 compounds, some hydrophilic and some lipophilic. While in vitro and in vivo measurements of human skin penetration of hydrophilic compounds generally agree, we know less about the relative penetration characteristics of lipophilic compounds in human subjects as against in vitro test systems using human skin. Modifications in methods for in vitro studies of lipophilic compounds include removal of the dermis from the skin preparation and the use of lipophilic receptor phase solution. These test methods have been applied in toxicology studies but have generally not been used to study lipophilic topical corticosteroids [42].

Metabolism of Corticosteroids

Metabolism of corticosteroids in the skin is yet another factor to consider as we evaluate new approaches to bioavailability testing. An important paper that prompted little follow-up when it was published in 1971 [43] now shows us the direction this research might take. In this study tritiated cortisol was applied to various skin sites in two human subjects and urinary excretion of metabolites was measured. Cortisol that was applied to the scrotum was excreted fairly rapidly as corticosteroid. However, cortisol that was applied to the abdomen, and that remained in the skin for a far longer period, was excreted primarily as oxysteroid. This result suggests that some areas of skin can extensively metabolize some corticosteroids before they reach their site of action, rendering them inactive. The investigator, Mavis Greaves, suggests that certain corticosteroids may owe their high potency to their ability to resist the effects of metabolizing enzymes in the skin. Investigators have been slow to follow up on these observations because of the difficulty of chemical analysis. However, now that HPLC is widely available, we will be able to examine and compare the metabolism of different corticosteroids. Ademola et al. [44] have demonstrated facile methods for quantifying the skin metabolism of xenobiotics.

Drug Partitioning in Normal and Diseased Skin

The ability to measure drug partitioning in different tissue compartments within the skin is an exciting development that will allow us to make precise determinations of topical corticosteroid pharmacokinetics within these compartments, rather than relying on crude measurements of throughput such as urinary excretion. There is now some evidence of differences between normal and diseased skin in the partitioning of topical corticosteroids, even when total absorption is the same.

In studies conducted in our laboratory, Wilhelm et al. [45] produced a model irritant contact dermatitis in guinea pigs by applying sodium lauryl sulfate to the skin. Topical formulations of 4 different ^{14}C-labeled agents with different pharmacochemical properties, each contained in the same vehicle, were then applied. In an in vitro experiment, the formulations were applied to guinea pig skin mounted on diffusion cells. Drug concentrations were higher in the diseased skin than in the control skin; and throughput of the 4 agents into the diffusion medium, an indicator of systemic absorption, was enhanced to an even greater degree in diseased skin. The enhancement of penetration in diseased skin was higher for the hydrophilic compounds (hydrocortisone, ibuprofen and indomethacin) than for the lipophilic compound (acitretin).

When the topical formulations were applied to living animals, partitioning varied for each of the agents. For hydrocortisone, stratum corneum drug concentrations were the same in irritated and normal skin, but measurements of dermal/epidermal drug levels in punch biopsy specimens showed 70% lower concentrations of hydrocortisone in diseased skin than in control skin. Systemic absorption of hydrocortisone, measured by 5-day urinary and fecal excretion, was higher in the animals with irritated skin than in controls [46].

Most of the human test models currently used to measure topical drug bioavailability – particularly the vasoconstrictor assay – are based on normal rather than diseased skin. Because the experimental evidence suggests that diseased skin may not interact in the same way with the complex delivery systems used in modern topical drug formulations, research should focus on developing additional models to measure topical drug pharmacokinetics in diseased skin. Furthermore, although drug throughput will remain valuable as a measure of systemic absorption, investigators will also need to develop ways to measure drug partitioning in the various tissue compartments of diseased skin [46].

Conclusions

Topical corticoids remain almost a panacea for many patients. The generations of improvement as summarized in our recent text have made many skin diseases far more manageable than with the first-generation hydrocortisone era [47]. Many valuable advances were empiric; today numerous theory-driven advances make us even more optimistic about the future.

References

1   Wester RC, Maibach HI: Dermatopharmacokinetics in clinical dermatology; in Bronaugh RL, Maibach HI (eds): Percutaneous Absorption. New York, Dekker, 1985, pp 125–132.
2   Rougier A, Dupuis D, Lotte C, Maibach HI: Stripping methods for measuring percutaneous absorption in vitro; in Bronaugh RL, Maibach HI (eds): Percutaneous Absorption. Mechanisms – Methods – Drug Delivery, ed 2. New York, Dekker, 1989, pp 415–434.
3   Wester RC, Noonan PK, Maibach HI: Percutaneous absorption of hydrocortisone increases with long-term administration: In vivo studies in the rhesus monkey. Arch Dermatol 1980;116:186–190.
4   Bucks DAW, Maibach HI, Guy RH: Percutaneous absorption of steroids: Effect of repeated application. J Pharm Sci 1985;74:1337–1339.
5   Bucks DAW, Maibach HI, Guy RH: In vivo percutaneous absorption: Effect of repeated application versus single dose; in Bronaugh RL, Maibach HI (eds): Percutaneous Absorption. Mechanisms – Methods – Drug Delivery, ed 2. New York, Dekker, 1989, pp 633–651.
6   Melendres JL, Bucks DAW, Camel E, Wester RC, Maibach HI: In vivo percutaneous absorption of hydrocortisone multiple application dosing in man. Pharm Res 1990;6:S–248.
7   McKenzie AW, Stoughton RB: Method for comparing percutaneous absorption of steroids. Arch Dermatol 1962;86:88–90.

8   Feldmann RJ, Maibach HI: Penetration of ^{14}C hydrocortisone through normal skin: The effect of stripping and occlusion. Arch Dermatol 1965;91:661–666.

9   Feldmann RJ, Maibach HI: Percutaneous penetration of steroids in man. J Invest Dermatol 1969; 52:89–94.

10   Wester RC, Noonan PK, Maibach HI: Frequency of application on percutaneous absorption of hydrocortisone. Arch Dermatol 1977;113:620–622.

11   Wester RC, Maibach HI: Relationship of topical dose and percutaneous absorption in rhesus monkey and man. J Invest Dermatol 1976;67:518–520.

12   Stoughton RB, Wullich K: The same glucocorticoid in brand-name products: Does increasing the concentration result in greater topical biological activity? Arch Dermatol 1989;125:1509–1511.

13   Feldmann RJ, Maibach HI: Regional variation in percutaneous penetration of ^{14}C cortisol in man. J Invest Dermatol 1967;48:181–183.

14   Guy RH, Maibach HI: Calculations of body exposure from percutaneous absorption data; in Bronaugh RL, Maibach HI (eds): Percutaneous Absorption. New York, Dekker, 1985, pp 461–466.

15   Wester RC, Maibach HI: In vivo percutaneous absorption; in Marzulli FN, Maibach HI (eds): Dermatotoxicology, ed 3. New York, Hemisphere, 1987, pp 135–152.

16   Wester RC, Bucks DAW, Maibach HI: In vivo percutaneous absorption of hydrocortisone in psoriatic patients and normal volunteers. J Am Acad Dermatol 1983;8:646–647.

17   Wester R, Mobayen M, Ryatt K, Bucks D, Maibach HI: In vivo percutaneous absorption of dithranol in psoriatic and normal volunteers; in Farber E (ed): Psoriasis. Amsterdam, Elsevier, 1987, p 429.

18   Wang JCT, Patel BG, Ehmann CW, Lowe N: The release and percutaneous permeation of anthralin products, using clinically involved and uninvolved psoriatic skin. J Am Acad Dermatol 1987;16: 812–821.

19   Schaefer H, Zesch A, Stüttgen G: Skin permeability; in Stüttgen G, Spier H, Schwarz E (eds): Normal and Pathologic Physiology of the Skin. Part III. Berlin, Springer, 1981, pp 795–802.

20   Schalla W, Jamoulle J-C, Schaefer H: Localization of compounds in different skin layers and its use as an indicator of percutaneous absorption; in Bronaugh RL, Maibach HI (eds): Percutaneous Absorption. Mechanisms – Methods – Drug Delivery, ed 2. New York, Dekker, 1989, pp 282–312.

21   Erlanger M, Martz GH, Ott F, Storck H, Rider J, Kessler S: Cutaneous absorption and urinary excretion of 6-^{14}C-5-fluorouracil ointment applied in an ointment to healthy and diseased human skin. Dermatologica 1970(suppl 1):7–14.

22   Foreman M, Clanchan I, Kelly I: The diffusion of nandrolone through occluded and non-occluded human skin. J Pharm Pharmacol 1978;30:152–157.

23   Shani J: Skin penetration of minerals in psoriatic and guinea pigs bathing in hypertonic salt solutions. Pharmacol Res Commun 1985;17:501–511.

24   Grice KA, Sattar H, Baker H: The cutaneous barrier to salts and water in psoriasis and in normal skin. Br J Dermatol 1973;88:459–463.

25   Bucks DAW, Maibach HI, Menczel E, Wester RC: Percutaneous penetration of hydrocortisone in humans following skin delipidization by 1:1 trichlorethane. Arch Dermatol Res 1983;275:242–245.

26   Bucks DAW, McMaster JR, Maibach HI, Guy RH: Bioavailability to topically administered steroids: A mass balance technique. J Invest Dermatol 1988;91:29–33.

27   Bronaugh RL, Weingarten DP, Lowe NJ: Differential rates of percutaneous absorption through the eczematous and normal skin of a monkey. J Invest Dermatol 1986;87:451–453.

28   Wester RC, Noonan PK, Maibach HI: Percutaneous absorption of hydrocortisone increases with long-term administration. Arch Dermatol 1980;116:186–188.

29   Turpeinen M: Influence of age and severity of dermatitis on the percutaneous absorption of hydrocortisone in children. Br J Dermatol 1988;118:517–522.

30   Turpeinen M, Mashkilleyson N, Bjorksten F, Salo OP: Percutaneous absorption of hydrocortisone during exacerbation and remission of atopic dermatitis in adults. Acta Derm Venereol (Stockh) 1988;68:331–335.

31   Moon KC, Wester RC, Maibach HI: Diseased skin models in the hairless guinea pig: In vivo percutaneous absorption. Dermatologica 1990;180:8–12.

32   Solomon AE, Lowe NJ: Percutaneous absorption in experimental epidermal disease. Arch Dermatol 1978;114:1029–1030.

33   Lambrey B, Schalla W, Kail N, Lahmy JP, Schaefer H: Influence of an essential fatty acid deficient diet on absorption of topical hydrocortisone in the rat. Br J Dermatol 1987;117:607–615.

34   Wilhelm K-P, Surber C, Maibach HI: Effect of sodium lauryl sulfate-induced skin irritation on in vitro percutaneous Absorption; in Bronaugh RL, Maibach HI (eds): In vitro Percutaneous Absorption: Principles, Fundamentals and Applications. Boca Raton, CRC Press, 1991, pp 265–273.

35   Moon KC, Maibach HI: Percutaneous absorption in diseased skin: Relationship to the exogenous dermatoses; in Menne T, Maibach HI (eds): Exogenous Dermatoses: Environmental Dermatitis. Boca Raton, CRC Press, 1991, pp 217–226.

36   Wester RC, Maibach HI: Percutaneous absorption in diseased skin; in Maibach HI, Surber C (eds): Topical Corticosteroids. Basel, Karger, 1992, pp 128–141.

37   Shah VP, Elkins J, Skelly JP: Relationship between in vivo skin blanching and in vitro release rate for betamethasone valerate creams. J Pharm Sci 1992;81:104–106.

38   Pershing LK, Silver BS, Krueger GG, Shah VP, Skelly JP: Feasibility of measuring the bioavailability of topical betamethasone formulations using drug content in skin and a skin blanching bioassay. Pharm Res 1992;9:45–51.

39   Wester RC, Maibach HI: In vivo animal models for percutaneous absorption; in Bronaugh RL, Maibach HI (eds): Percutaneous Absorption. Mechanisms – Methods – Drug Delivery, ed 2. New York, Dekker, 1989, pp 221–238.

40   Bartek MJ, LaBudde JA, Maibach HI: Skin permeability in vivo: Comparison in rat, pig, and man. J Invest Dermatol 1972;58:114–123.

41   Bronaugh RL: Determination of percutaneous absorption by in vitro techniques; in Bronaugh RL, Maibach HI (eds): Percutaneous Absorption. Mechanisms – Methods – Drug Delivery, ed 2. New York, Dekker, 1989, pp 239–258.

42   Bronaugh RL, Collier SW: In vivo-in vitro correlations for hydrophobic compound; in Bronaugh RL, Maibach HI (eds): In vitro Percutaneous Absorption: Principles, Fundamentals and Applications. Boca Raton, CRC Press, 1991, pp 199–205.

43   Greaves MS: The in vivo catabolism of cortisol by human skin. J Invest Dermatol 1971;57:100–107.

44   Ademola J, Wester R, Maibach HI: Cutaneous metabolism of theophylline by the human skin. J Invest Dermatol 1992;98:310–314.

45   Wilhelm K-P, Surber C, Maibach HI: Effect of sodium lauryl sulfate-induced skin irritation on in vitro percutaneous absorption of four drugs. J Invest Dermatol 1991;96:963–967.

46   Wilhelm K-P, Surber C, Maibach HI: Effect of sodium lauryl sulfate-induced skin irritation on in vivo percutaneous absorption penetration of four drugs. J Invest Dermatol 1991;97:927–932.

47   Maibach H, Surber C (eds): Topical Corticosteroids. Basel, Karger, 1992.

Ronald C. Wester, Department of Dermatology, University of California,
School of Medicine, Box 0989, Surge 110, San Francisco, CA 94143–0989 (USA)

Korting HC, Maibach HI (eds): Topical Glucocorticoids with Increased Benefit/Risk Ratio.
Curr Probl Dermatol. Basel, Karger, 1993, vol 21, pp 61–66

....

Metabolism of Topical Drugs within the Skin, in Particular Glucocorticoids

Kiyoshi Kubota, John Ademola, Howard I. Maibach

Department of Dermatology, University of California at San Francisco,
School of Medicine, San Francisco, Calif., USA

Several models have been developed to study skin metabolism. They include the skin-flap technique [1], the 'dynamic' culture system [2] and the living skin equivalent (LSE) [3, 4]. The LSE, constructed from cultured human epidermal cells and fibroblasts, has three layers which are equivalent to the stratum corneum, viable epidermis and dermis, respectively [3, 4]. In the present study, the metabolism of betamethasone 17-valerate in homogenized LSE is examined as a first step to the 'simultaneous diffusion and metabolism' experiment [5].

Materials and Methods

Degradation of Betamethasone 17-Valerate in Homogenates of Living Skin Equivalent
The LSE, Testskin™ (diameter ~2 cm), with a standard 6-well plate and culture medium, was a generous gift from Organogenesis (Cambridge, Mass., USA). Methods for preparing LSE and relevant information have been published earlier [3, 4].

A 4-μg/ml betamethasone 17-valerate solution was prepared immediately before the experiment by adding 50 μl of 16 mg/ml of betamethasone 17-valerate in ethanol to 200 ml of culture medium. The homogenates of 4 LSE pieces were suspended in 80 ml of this solution. One-milliliter samples of these solutions were transferred into small vials and incubated at 37 °C in the tissue culture incubator for 40 min to 48 h. Samples were collected in duplicate. Immediately after the collection of each 1-ml sample, 50 μl of a 40-μg/ml prednisone solution in methanol, as internal standard, and 3 ml of 2% methanol in dichloromethane were added. The mixture was then vortexed for 1 min. After centrifugation at 3,000 rpm for 5 min, the upper aqueous phase was discarded. The organic phase was filtered using a column packed with diatomaceous earth, Celite 545® (Manville, Denver, Colo., USA), and evaporated to dryness. The sample was reconstituted in 2% methanol in dichlor-

Table 1. First and second degradation steps of betamethasone 17-valerate

---

Betamethasone 17-valerate

$\downarrow$ k_1 *isomerization*

Betamethasone 21-valerate

$\downarrow$ k_2 *hydrolysis*

Betamethasone

The first step is not affected by enzyme but the second step is accelerated by esterase.

---

omethane and injected into the chromatograph. Corticosteroids were measured by a normal-phase HPLC method using a Rabbit-HP constant flow pump (Rainin Instruments, Berkeley, Calif., USA), a Knauer variable wavelength ultraviolet detector (Spektralphotometer, Nr. 731.87, Bad Homburg, FRG) set at 240 nm and an integrator, Shimadzu Chromatopac (CR 601, Kyoto, Japan). A silica gel column, LiChrosorb Si-100, 10 µm, 250 × 4 mm internal diameter (Merck, Darmstadt, FRG), was used for compound separation. The chromatographic solvent system consisted of 0.1% water, 4.5% methanol and 30% dichloromethane in *n*-hexane. The flow rate was 2 ml/min. The retention times for betamethasone 21-valerate, betamethasone 17-valerate, prednisone (internal standard) and betamethasone were 3.2, 3.9, 7.7 and 11.4 min, respectively. Detection limits were 5 ng per sample (signal to noise ratio of 4:1) for all of the measured compounds. Recoveries of corticosteroids from the culture medium were greater than 96%.

Compartment Model for the Degradation of Betamethasone 17-Valerate in Skin Homogenate

The amount and concentration of the three corticosteroids, betamethasone 17-valerate, betamethasone 21-valerate and betamethasone, are expressed as the value equivalent to betamethasone 17-valerate throughout the study. Conversions from betamethasone 17-valerate to betamethasone 21-valerate and from betamethasone 21-valerate to betamethasone (table 1) were assumed to be first-order [6, 7], such that:

$$\frac{dC_{b17}}{dt} = -k_1 \, C_{b17}, \tag{1}$$

$$\frac{dC_{b21}}{dt} = k_1 \, C_{b17} - k_2 \, C_{b21} \text{ and} \tag{2}$$

$$\frac{dC_b}{dt} = k_2 \, C_{b21}, \tag{3}$$

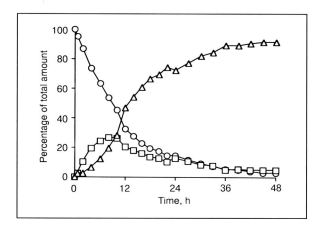

Fig. 1. Mean (n = 2) percentage of total amount of beta-methasone 17-valerate (○), betamethasone 21-valerate (□) and betamethasone (△) versus time in culture medium without skin homogenate when 4 μg/ml (final concentration) of betamethasone 17-valerate was added at t = 0 h.

where C_{b17}, C_{b21} and C_b are the concentrations of betamethasone 17-valerate, betametha-sone 21-valerate and betamethasone, respectively. The first-order degradation constants, k_1 and k_2, were estimated by the nonlinear least-squares method.

Results

No significant peaks indicating possible metabolites of betamethasone appeared when the chromatograph was carefully traced until 150 min after the sample injection. The mean (± SD, n = 21 each) total amount of the three cortico-steroids, betamethasone 17-valerate, betamethasone 21-valerate and betametha-sone, in the samples without skin homogenate and in those with skin homogenate were 3.86 ± 0.17 μg (96.5 ± 4.3%) and 3.15 ± 0.50 μg (78.8 ± 12.5%), respec-tively, when measured at the 21 different occasions between 40 min and 48 h. No correlation between the recovery from the samples with skin homogenate and sampling time was observed; e.g., the recoveries were 3.14, 3.32, 2.82, 3.10 and 2.86 μg at 40 min, 12 h, 24 h, 36 h and 48 h, respectively.

When the percentage of each compound was plotted versus time course, the betamethasone 17-valerate versus time profiles without skin homogenate (fig. 1) were essentially identical to those with skin homogenate (fig. 2). On the other

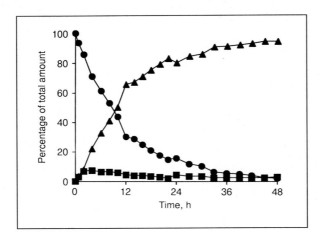

Fig. 2. Mean (n = 2) percentage of total amount of beta-methasone 17-valerate (●), betamethasone 21-valerate (■) and betamethasone (▲) versus time in culture medium with skin homogenate when 4 µg/ml (final concentration) of betamethasone 17-valerate was added at t = 0 h.

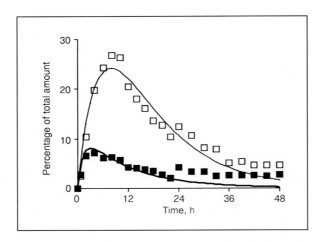

Fig. 3. Computer-generated profiles of percentage of total amount of betamethasone 21-valerate (solid lines) according to equations 1–3 and observed values (□, ■). Closed symbols represent time courses in culture medium with skin homogenate while open symbols indicate those without skin homogenate.

Table 2. First-order degradation rate constants of betamethasone 17-valerate at $37\,°C$ in culture medium

Culture medium	k_1 h^{-1}	k_2 h^{-1}
With skin homogenate	0.0837	0.797
Without skin homogenate	0.0843	0.178

k_1 = First-order degradation rate constant from betamethasone 17-valerate to betamethasone 21-valerate; k_2 = first-order degradation rate constant from betamethasone 21-valerate to betamethasone.

hand, the fraction of betamethasone 21-valerate was larger and that of betamethasone was smaller in the samples without skin homogenate (fig. 1) than in those with homogenate (fig. 2), particularly in the early phase. Equations 1–3 generally adequately modeled the data observed with or without skin homogenate. However, a deviation of the percentage of betamethasone 21-valerate from the model prediction occurred after 24 h in the samples with skin homogenate (fig. 3). Table 2 shows the corresponding k_1 and k_2 values. The half-lives of betamethasone 17-valerate in the culture medium at $37\,°C$ were 8.3 and 8.2 h with and without the LSE homogenate, respectively.

Discussion

The average total amount of betamethasone 17-valerate, betamethasone 21-valerate and betamethasone extracted from the samples with skin homogenate approximated $3.15\,\mu g$. There was no correlation between the total amount recovered and the sampling interval, and the chromatographic profile did not suggest metabolite formation. Therefore, incomplete compound extraction, rather than further metabolism from betamethasone, probably accounted for the loss. Indeed, when the percentage of each corticosteroid was plotted as a function of time, betamethasone 17-valerate versus time profiles were almost identical to each other with or without skin homogenate (fig. 1, 2). This observation is compatible with a previous report [7] where the transformation of betamethasone 17-valerate to betamethasone 21-valerate was essentially irreversible (25 times faster than that of betamethasone 21-valerate to betamethasone 17-valerate) and those changes were not influenced by esterase. There are agreements between the k_1 value (table 2) and the value previously reported [7]. On the other hand, the conversion of betamethasone 21-valerate to betamethasone was accelerated when skin homogenate was incorporated (table 2; fig. 1, 2).

In the samples with the LSE homogenate, the percentage of betamethasone 21-valerate after 24 h was always larger than the theoretical value assuming that the k_2 value is constant (fig. 3). Therefore, the esterase activity may be decreased or lost after 24 h in the LSE homogenate when suspended in the culture medium.

In conclusion, LSE has a sufficient level of esterase to induce a discernible change in the conversion of betamethasone 21-valerate to betamethasone. The conversion of betamethasone 17-valerate to betamethasone 21-valerate was not affected by the skin homogenate, which is in agreement with the previous report [7].

References

1   Carver MP, Levi PE, Riviere JE: Parathion metabolism during percutaneous absorption in perfused porcine skin. Pest Biochem Physiol 1990;38:245–254.
2   Kao J, Hall J: Skin absorption and cutaneous first pass metabolism of topical steroids: In vitro studies with mouse skin in organ culture. J Pharmacol Exp Ther 1987;241:482–487.
3   Bell E, Parenteau N, Gay R, Nolte C, Kemp P, Bilbo P, Ekstein B, Johnson E: The living skin equivalent: Its manufacture, its organotypic properties and its responses to irritants. Toxicol In Vitro 1991;5:591–596.
4   Parenteau NL, Nolte CM, Bilbo P, Rosenberg M, Wilkins LM, Johnson EW, Watson S, Mason VS, Bell E: Epidermis generated in vitro: Practical considerations and applications. J Cell Biochem 1991;45:245–251.
5   Liu P, Higuchi WI, Ghanem A-H, Kurihara-Bergstrom T, Good WR: Quantitation of simultaneous diffusion and metabolism of β-estradiol in hairless mouse skin: Enzyme distribution and intrinsic diffusion/metabolism parameters. Int J Pharmacol 1990;64:7–25.
6   Yip YW, Po ALW: The stability of betamethasone-17-valerate in semi-solid bases. J Pharm Pharmacol 1979;31:400–402.
7   Cheung YW, Po ALW, Irwin WJ: Cutaneous biotransformation as a parameter in the modulation of the activity of topical corticosteroids. Int J Pharmacol 1985;26:175–189.

Kiyoshi Kubota, MD, Department of Dermatology,
University of California at San Francisco, School of Medicine, San Francisco, CA 94143 (USA)

Korting HC, Maibach HI (eds): Topical Glucocorticoids with Increased Benefit/Risk Ratio.
Curr Probl Dermatol. Basel, Karger, 1993, vol 21, pp 67–72

....

Influence of Glucocorticoids on the Epidermal Langerhans Cell

A. Mieke Mommaas

Department of Dermatology, University Hospital Leiden, The Netherlands

Langerhans cells (LCs) constitute only 2–4% of the epidermal cells, but they play an important role in the immune responses in the skin [1]. They have a dendritic configuration, are of bone marrow origin and express membrane ATPase, FC-IgG and C3b receptors, CD1a/T6 antigen and S-100 protein, and are the only cells in normal epidermis that express MHC class II molecules (Ia in mice and HLA class II in man). The role of epidermal LCs in antigen presentation was first established in 1973 by Silberberg [2] and is now well documented [3], with LCs having a key role in the pathogenesis of allergic contact dermatitis. Topical glucocorticoids are the agents most commonly used for the treatment of inflammatory skin disorders and inhibit not only the elicitation phase, but also the induction phase of allergic contact dermatitis [4–6]. During both the induction and the elicitation phase, LCs present antigen on their cell surface in the context of MHC class II molecules. There is ample evidence that topical glucocorticoid therapy decreases the density of MHC-class-II-positive LCs in the epidermis [7–11]. However, in all these studies LCs were identified by immunofluorescence staining of surface markers, making it impossible to determine whether the cells were destroyed or whether they had lost their surface antigens. Electron microscopy can solve this problem, since at the ultrastructural level LCs can be easily recognized by their unique cytoplasmic organelle, the Birbeck granule. We have used a highly sensitive immunoelectron-microscopic technique to study the effect of topical steroids on human epidermal LCs, using a colloidal-gold-labeled anti-

HLA class II antibody. This method allows both the recognition of LCs and the expression of HLA class II molecules on these cells on the same specimen. Using this method we studied the effect on normal LCs and on LCs of an active psoriasis lesion, a condition in which LCs are stimulated.

Materials and Methods

Subjects and Treatment

Two healthy volunteers and one psoriasis patient were included in the study. The volunteers applied glucocorticoid ointment to localized areas of the right buttock twice daily for 7 days. One applied hydrocortisone 1%, the other clobetasol propionate 0.05% (Dermovate®). 4-mm punch biopsies were obtained from the left, untreated buttock and from the right, treated buttock. The psoriasis patient was treated with triamcinolone acetonide 0.1% twice daily. 4-mm punch biopsies were obtained from involved skin prior to and 7 days after treatment.

Immunoelectron Microscopy

The biopsies were processed for immunoelectron microscopy as described elsewhere [12]. Briefly, immediately after biopsy, the specimens were immersed in fixative (2% paraformaldehyde in phosphate buffer) and cut into small blocks which were kept in the same fixative for at least 18 h. Then the specimens were cryoprotected by 2.3 M sucrose and frozen in liquid nitrogen. Ultrathin cryosections were prepared and incubated with a monoclonal anti-HLA class II antibody (PdV 5.2, kindly provided by Dr. F. Koning, Leiden, The Netherlands) conjugated to 10-nm colloidal gold. After incubation procedures, the sections were embedded in methylcellulose, stained with uranyl acetate and viewed with a Philips EM 410 electron microscope.

Results

In normal, unstimulated epidermal LCs, HLA class II molecules, visualized by 10-nm colloidal gold particles, were present in membrane-limited, electron-dense, intracellular vesicles, representing late endosomes and/or lysosomes [13] (fig. 1a). Upon 7 days of steroid treatment, this pattern of HLA class II expression was not changed (fig. 1b, showing the results of the volunteer who applied hydrocortisone; the results with clobetasol propionate were similar; data not shown). In a psoriasis lesion, LCs are stimulated. This resulted in an enhanced cell surface HLA class II expression on the epidermal LCs (fig. 1c). This enhanced cell surface expression was not modulated by topical treatment with triamcinolone for 7 days (fig. 1d).

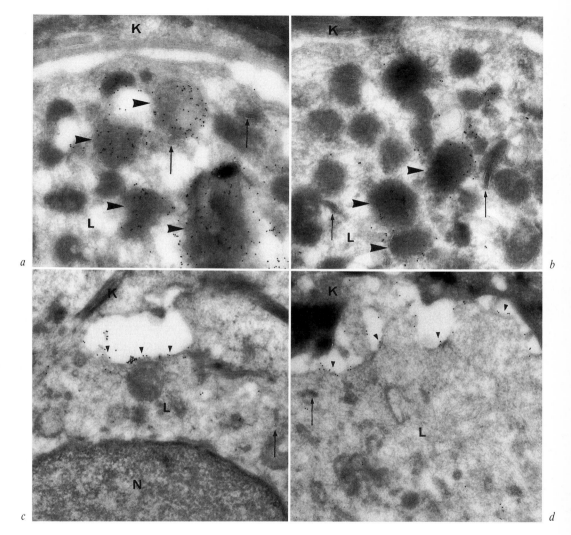

Fig. 1. Details of epidermal LCs in ultracryosections of human skin, incubated with the monoclonal anti-HLA class II antibody PdV 5.2, conjugated to 10-nm colloidal gold. *a* In normal skin, with gold particles predominantly in intracellular electron-dense vesicles (large arrowheads). *b* After topical treatment with hydrocortisone 1% for 7 days, showing no differences in comparison to normal LCs. *c* In an active psoriasis lesion without treatment, showing enhanced cell surface HLA class II labeling (small arrowheads). *d* In a psoriasis lesion, treated with triamcinolone acetonide 0.1% for 7 days, showing no differences with LCs prior to treatment. Arrows point to Birbeck granules. K = Keratinocyte; L = Langerhans cell; N = nucleus. ×32,500.

Discussion

Several reports have compared both the effect of glucocorticoids and ultra-violet B light on epidermal LCs, and it was shown that both physicochemical agents reduce the local density of LCs which stain for ATPase activity and MHC class II antigen [11, 14]; this reduction was paralleled by a decrease in functional activity. The present study shows that topical glucocorticoids do not influence the expression of HLA class II molecules on human epidermal LCs. We previously examined the ultrastructural localization of HLA class II molecules during allergic contact dermatitis and the influence of ultraviolet B on these antigens [12, and unpubl. data]. Furthermore, we studied the influence of long-term ultraviolet B and PUVA therapy on the LC expression of HLA class II antigens [unpubl. data]. We showed that, similar as after glucocorticoid application, ultraviolet light did not alter the localization of HLA class II molecules on LCs as compared to normal, unstimulated LCs. This would be in keeping with Furue and Katz [15], who reported that in vitro treatment of murine epidermal cells with glucocorticoids results in a dose- and time-dependent fall in the number of Ia-positive cells, but that residual Ia-positive LCs express normal amounts of Ia antigen on a cell-for-cell basis, indicating that a subgroup of LCs is resistant to the deleterious effects of glucocorticoids. Ashworth et al. [16] demonstrated a similar subgroup of steroid-resistant LCs in human skin. They suggested that this apparent steroid resistance may reflect heterogeneity in the density of expression of LC steroid receptors, but a recent report could not detect any glucocorticoid receptors on human epidermal LCs [17]. We only found HLA-class-II-positive and no HLA-class-II-negative LCs, which means that we could not confirm the existence of such a resistance to topical glucocorticoids. This discrepancy may be explained by the use of different experimental techniques: Furue and Katz [15] and Ashworth et al. [16] used isolated epidermal cells while we applied antibodies on sections of whole tissue. Isolation procedures such as trypsin treatment can cause changes or destruction of membrane components.

In both the healthy volunteers and the psoriasis patient, we counted the number of LCs before and after glucocorticoid treatment. Quantification was performed at the ultrastructural level, and LCs were identified by specific morphological features such as Birbeck granules, and not by cell surface markers that can be affected by glucocorticoids. We did not find a reduction in the number of LCs after steroid treatment, but since the number of subjects that we investigated was low, conclusive data are not available yet. Decrease of LCs by cytotoxic effects of glucocorticoids cannot be ruled out, although we did not find LCs that showed signs of destruction.

At present it is not clear why glucocorticoids impair the function of epidermal LCs, although there are several theories about the mechanisms that are responsible. It has been shown that for allostimulation of T cells the mere presence of cell surface Ia antigens on rat or murine leukocytes is not sufficient [18, 19]. Furthermore, there is ample evidence that ultraviolet irradiation and glucocorticoid treatment of the skin alter the profile of cytokines and adhesion molecules, and these substances are well known to play an important role in immunological functions of the skin [20–26]. Modulatory effects of glucocorticoids on these factors need further investigation.

References

1 Streilein JW, Bergstresser PR: Langerhans cells: Antigen presenting cells of the epidermis. Immunobiology 1984;168:285–300.
2 Silberberg I: Apposition of mononuclear cells to Langerhans cells in allergic reactions: An ultrastructural study. Acta Derm Venereol (Stockh) 1973;53:1–12.
3 Stingl G, Tamaki K, Katz SI: Origin and function of epidermal Langerhans cells. Immunol Rev 1980;53:149–174.
4 Burrows WM, Stoughton RB: Inhibition of induction of human contact sensitization by topical glucocorticosteroids. Arch Dermatol 1976;112:175–178.
5 Lynch DH, Gurish MF, Daynes RA: Relationship between epidermal Langerhans cell density, ATPase activity and the induction of contact hypersensitivity. J Immunol 1981;126:1892–1897.
6 Prens EP, Benne K, Geursen-Reitsma AM, van Dijk G, Benner R, van Joost Th: Effects of topically applied glucocorticosteroids on patch test responses and recruitment of inflammatory cells in allergic contact dermatitis. Agents Actions 1989;26:125–127.
7 Nordlund JJ, Ackles AE, Lerner AB: The effects of ultraviolet light and certain drugs on Ia bearing Langerhans cells in murine epidermis. Cell Immunol 1981;60:50–63.
8 Belsito DV, Flotte TJ, Lim HW, Baer RL, Thorbecke GJ, Gigli I: Effects of glucocorticoids on epidermal Langerhans cells. J Exp Med 1982;155:291–302.
9 Berman B, France DS, Martinelli GP, Hess A: Modulation of expression of epidermal Langerhans cell properties following in situ exposure to glucocorticosteroids. J Invest Dermatol 1983;80:168–171.
10 Belsito DV, Baer RL, Thorbecke GJ, Gigli I: Effect of glucocorticosteroids and gamma irradiation on epidermal Langerhans cells. J Invest Dermatol 1984;82:136–138.
11 Aberer W, Romani N, Elbe A, Stingl G: Effects of physicochemical agents on murine epidermal Langerhans cells and Thy-1-positive dendritic epidermal cells. J Immunol 1986;136:1210–1216.
12 Mommaas AM, Wijsman MC, Mulder AA, van Praag MCG, Vermeer BJ, Koning F: HLA class II expression on human epidermal Langerhans cells in situ: Upregulation during allergic contact dermatitis. Hum Immunol 1992;34:99–106.
13 Neefjes JJ, Ploegh HL: Intracellular transport of MHC class II molecules. Immunol Today 1992;13:179–184.
14 Belsito DV, Baer RL, Gigli I, Thorbecke GJ: Effect of combined topical glucocorticoids and ultraviolet B irradiation on epidermal Langerhans cells. J Invest Dermatol 1984;83:347–351.
15 Furue M, Katz SI: Direct effects of glucocorticosteroids on epidermal Langerhans cells. J Invest Dermatol 1989;92:342–347.
16 Ashworth J, Kahan MC, Breatnach SM: Flow cytometrically-sorted residual HLA-DR+T6+ Langerhans cells in topical steroid-treated human skin express normal amounts of HLA-DR and CD1a/T6 antigens and exhibit normal alloantigen presenting capacity. J Invest Dermatol 1989;92:258–262.
17 Serres M, Viac J, Schmitt D, Thivolet J: Glucocorticoid receptor expression in human epidermal cells. J Invest Dermatol 1992;98:523.
18 Klinkert WEF, La Badie J, Bowers WE: Accessory and stimulating properties of dendritic cells and macrophages isolated from various rat tissues. J Exp Med 1982;156:1–19.

19 Sunshine GH, Katz Dr, Czitrom AA: Heterogeneity of stimulator cells in the murine mixed leuko-cyte response. Eur J Immunol 1982;12:9–15.

20 Ansel JC, Luger TA, Green I: The effect of in vitro and in vivo UV irradiation on the production of ETAF activity by human and murine keratinocytes. J Invest Dermatol 1983;81:519–523.

21 Gahring L, Baltz M, Pepys MB, Daynes R: Effect of ultraviolet radiation on production of epider-mal cell thymocyte-activating factor/interleukin 1 in vivo and in vitro. Proc Natl Acad Sci USA 1984;81:1189–1202.

22 Kupper TS, Chua AO, Flood P, McGuire J, Gubler U: Interleukin 1 gene expression in cultured human keratinocytes is augmented by ultraviolet irradiation. J Clin Invest 1987;80:430–436.

23 Kirnbauer R, Köck A, Neuner P, Förster E, Krutmann J, Urbanski A, Schaur E, Ansel JC, Schwarz T, Luger TA: Regulation of epidermal cell interleukin-6 production by UV light and corticosteroids. J Invest Dermatol 1991;96:484–489.

24 Lee SW, Morhenn VB, Ilnicka J, Eugui EM, Allison AC: Autocrine stimulation of interleukin-1α and transforming growth factor α production in human keratinocytes and its antagonism by gluco-corticoids. J Invest Dermatol 1991;97:106–110.

25 Krutmann J, Köck A, Schaur E, Parlow F, Möller A, Kapp A, Förster E, Schöpf E, Luger FA: Tumor necrosis factor β and ultraviolet radiation are potent regulators of human keratinocyte ICAM-1 expression. J Invest Dermatol 1990;95:127–131.

26 Sawami MK, Lyons MB, Rothlein PR, Norris DA: Study of the effects of corticosteroids and reti-noids on induction of ICAM-1 on cultured human keratinocytes. J Invest Dermatol 1989;92:512.

A. Mieke Mommaas, PhD, Department of Dermatology, Bldg. 1H, Hl-Q,
University Hospital Leiden, PO Box 9600, NL–2300 RC Leiden (The Netherlands)

Korting HC, Maibach HI (eds): Topical Glucocorticoids with Increased Benefit/Risk Ratio.
Curr Probl Dermatol. Basel, Karger, 1993, vol 21, pp 73–78

....

Effect of Glucocorticosteroids on Number and Function of Connective-Tissue Cells

R. Hein

Dermatologische Klinik der Universität Regensburg, BRD

Corticosteroids are very potent drugs that are used in many acute and chronic skin diseases. However, their long-term application often induces profound side effects. Besides the well-known systemic complications, local application of corticosteroids often leads to skin atrophy, delayed wound healing and/or striae distensae [1]. The basis of this phenomenon has been intensively investigated in recent years [2–5].

It is well established that corticosteroids can inhibit cell proliferation and mitosis [6], decrease collagen [7] and glycosaminoglycan synthesis [8], and have an inhibitory effect on general protein production. There is consensus that corticosteroids directly influence the metabolism of dermal fibroblasts. Corticosteroids can also interfere indirectly with the biosynthetic capacities of fibroblasts. This is due to the fact that corticosteroids affect the inflammatory system and inhibit the migration of inflammatory cells during inflammatory reactions.

Therefore, we wished to use in vitro systems which allow to examine the influence of various drugs on the biosynthetic capacities of fibroblasts and to obtain data concerning both newly developed nonhalogenated corticosteroids and conventional fluorinated corticosteroids.

Influence of Corticosteroids on Cell Growth and Morphology

Corticosteroids have been shown to act as modulators of cell proliferation, which can either inhibit or stimulate DNA synthesis and cell growth, both in primary culture or in established cell lines [7]. In our system, corticosteroids added to fibroblast cultures showed a strong dosage-dependent influence on the

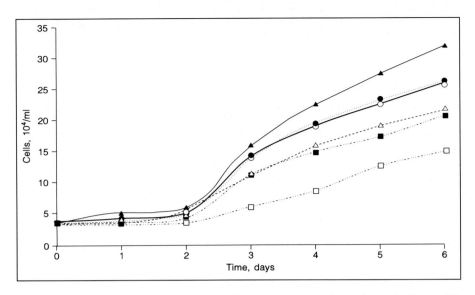

Fig. 1. Inhibition of proliferation of fibroblast cultures by various corticosteroids (10^{-5} *M*): □ = desoximethasone; ■ = betamethasone 17-valerate; △ = prednicarbate; ● = hydrocortisone; ○ = hydrocortisone buteprate; ▲ = control. The cells were seeded at low density (3×10^4 cells/ml) and duplicate cultures were counted daily.

proliferation of cells [for details, cf. ref. 9]. The fluorinated corticosteroids desoximethasone and betamethasone 17-valerate (10^{-5} *M*) reduced the rate of proliferation to about 50% of the controls, while the nonhalogenated substances were less active (fig. 1). Alteration in cell morphology (checked by phase-contrast microscopy; fig. 2) was noted when high concentrations of halogenated corticosteroids were used. These results were corroborated when cell viability was checked by the trypan blue test (table 1).

Ethanol used as solvent for the corticosteroids was added to the medium of fibroblasts in various concentrations and did not reveal any effect on cell growth, morphology or chemotactic response.

Influence of Corticosteroids on Chemotactic Activity of Fibroblasts

Chemotaxis, the directional migration of cells towards a gradient, is thought to play an important role in many biological processes such as inflammation, fibrosis and wound healing, as well as during tissue remodelling [10]. In order to

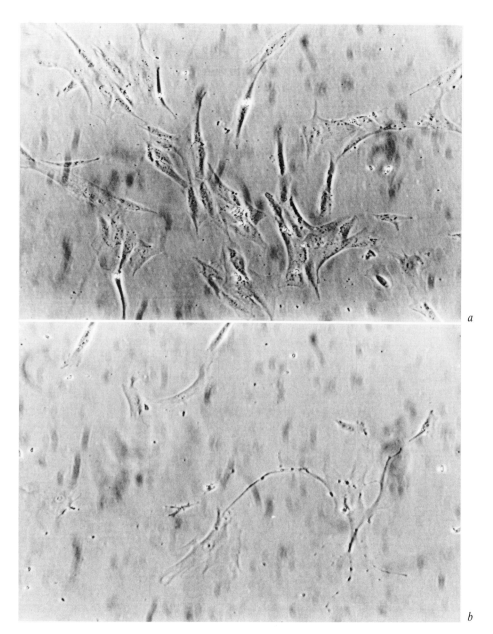

a

b

Fig. 2. Phase-contrast microphotography of fibroblasts after 3 days in culture *(a)*: typical asteroid configuration. Parallel cultures were treated with betamethasone 17-valerate (10^{-5} *M*; *b*): rarefication and thinning of cells. Cells treated with nonhalogenated derivatives did not show any alteration of morphology.

Table 1. Cell viability checked by the trypan blue test, expressed as relative proportion of dead cells

Corticosteroid	Day 1	Day 6
Control	6	10
Hydrocortisone	16	19
Hydrocortisone buteprate	12	20
Prednicarbate	8	19
Betamethasone 17-valerate	20	32
Desoximethasone	22	31

investigate the influence of different corticosteroids on these biological events, chemotaxis was studied in blind well Boyden chambers [11]. Fibroblast conditioned medium was used as chemoattractant [12]. Preincubation of cells with various corticosteroids either for 3 days or added prior to the assay (4 h) resulted in a marked decrease in chemotactic response of fibroblasts when high concentrations (10^{-5} M) of corticosteroids were used (fig. 3). However, when the cells were incubated with low concentrations of corticosteroids (10^{-9} M) there was a dissociation of their influence on the chemotactic response. Only the fluorinated substances (desoximethasone, betamethasone 17-valerate) showed a marked decrease in the chemotactic response, while the nonhalogenated corticosteroids (prednicarbate, hydrocortisone, hydrocortisone buteprate) showed only slight inhibition (fig. 3).

Discussion

Corticosteroids are known to reveal a strong anti-inflammatory activity, but also to inhibit the metabolism of many cell types. Recently, substances have been developed which are thought to show less side effects. We, therefore, intended to use different in vitro systems to characterize the response of fibroblasts to these agents.

High concentrations of fluorinated corticosteroids (10^{-5} M, betamethasone 17-valerate, desoximethasone) affected the viability of the cells as detected by the trypan blue test and altered the morphology. The logarithmic growth of fibroblasts was markedly inhibited when high concentrations (10^{-5} M) of corticosteroids were added to the cultures. Also consistent with previous observations, synthesis of noncollagenous proteins was inhibited by most of the corticosteroids used [11].

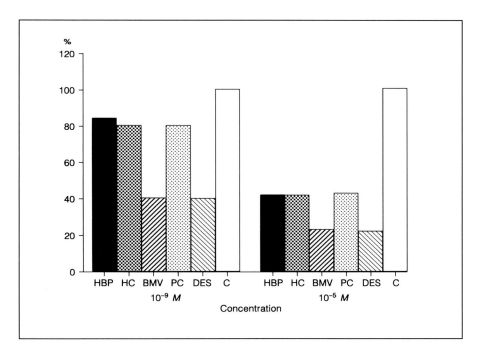

Fig. 3. Influence of corticosteroids on chemotactic response of fibroblasts. Cells were exposed for 3 days to various corticosteroids in concentrations of 10^{-9} and 10^{-5} *M*. The chemotactic activity is expressed as a percentage of corresponding activity of untreated cultures (100%). HBP = Hydrocortisone buteprate; HC = hydrocortisone; BMV = betamethasone 17-valerate; PC = prednicarbate; DES = desoximethasone; C = control.

The chemotactic response of fibroblasts to various chemoattractants, representing another function of these cells, is thought to control the formation of repair tissue during wound healing and is probably also important for the continuous remodelling of connective tissue [10]. Corticosteroids were shown to reduce chemotaxis of fibroblasts without influencing random migration. Reduced chemotaxis was found to be affected even at low concentrations of potent corticosteroids and might therefore play an important role to explain delayed wound healing which is often observed during systemic or local treatment with corticosteroids.

Inhibition of the migration of fibroblasts could also play a role together with reduced collagen and protein synthesis in the development of atrophy following long-term application of topical corticosteroids. Most of the effects of corticosteroids on the metabolism of fibroblasts were dose-dependent. However, when different derivatives were compared, fluorinated compounds were found to be most active in affecting fibroblast metabolism.

It remains to be seen whether nonhalogenated corticosteroids are internalized into the cell to a lesser extent than the fluorinated derivatives under in vitro conditions or whether the data indicate a dissociation of the inflammatory activity and inhibition of the biosynthetic capacities of fibroblasts.

References

1   Cutroneo KR, Rokowski R, Counts DF: Glucocorticoid and collagen synthesis: Comparison of in vivo and cell culture studies. Collagen Relat Res 1981;1:557–568.
2   Kivirikko KI, Laitinen O, Aer J, Halme J: Studies with ^{14}C-proline on the action of cortisone on the metabolism of collagen in the rat. Biochem Pharmacol 1965;14:1445–1451.
3   Bauer EA, Kronberger A, Valle KJ, Jeffrey J, Eisen AZ: Glucocorticoid modulation of collagenase expression in human skin fibroblast cultures: Evidence of pretranslational inhibition. Biochim Biophys Acta 1985;825:227–235.
4   Ponec M: Effects of glucocorticosteroids on cultured skin fibroblasts and keratinocytes. Int J Dermatol 1984;23:11–24.
5   Uitto J, Mustakallio KK: Effect of hydrocortisone acetate, fluocinolone acetonide, fluclorolone acetamide, betamethasone-17-valerate and fluprednyliden-21-acetate on collagen biosynthesis. Biochem Pharmacol 1971;20:2495–2503.
6   Ponec M, Haasper I, Viaden GD, Bachra B: Effect of glucocorticosteroids on primary human skin fibroblasts. II. Effect on total protein and collagen biosynthesis by confluent cell cultures. Arch Dermatol Res 1977;259:125–134.
7   Ponec M, de Haas C, Bachra BN, Polano MK: Effects of glucocorticosteroids on primary human skin fibroblasts. I. Inhibition of the proliferation of cultured primary human skin and mouse L-929 fibroblasts. Arch Dermatol Res 1977;259:117–124.
8   Särnstrand B, Brattsand R, Malmström A: Effect of glucocorticoids on glycosaminoglycan metabolism in cultured human skin fibroblasts. J Invest Dermatol 1982;79:412–417.
9   Hein R, Korting HC, Mehring T: Differential effect of medium potent non-halogenated double-ester type and conventional glucocorticoids on proliferation and chemotaxis of fibroblasts in vitro. Skin Pharmacol; in press.
10 Grotendorst GR, Martin GR: Cell movements in wound healing and fibrosis; in Schattenkirchner M (ed): Rheumatology. Basel, Karger, 1986, vol 10: Connective Tissue – Biological and Clinical Aspects; Kühn K, Krieg Th (vol eds), pp 385–403.
11 Hein R, Mauch C, Hatamochi A, Krieg Th: Influence of corticosteroids on chemotactic response and collagen metabolism of human skin fibroblasts. Biochem Pharmacol 1988;37:2723–2729.
12 Mensing H, Pontz B, Müller PK, Gauss-Müller V: A study on fibroblast chemotaxis using conditioned medium and fibronectin as chemoattractants. Eur J Cell Biol 1983;29:268–273.

Dr. med. Rüdiger Hein, Dermatologische Klinik der Universität Regensburg,
Franz-Josef-Strauss-Allee 11, D–93053 Regensburg (FRG)

Korting HC, Maibach HI (eds): Topical Glucocorticoids with Increased Benefit/Risk Ratio.
Curr Probl Dermatol. Basel, Karger, 1993, vol 21, pp 79–88

....

Topical Tretinoin Prevents Corticosteroid-Induced Atrophy without Lessening the Anti-Inflammatory Effect

Lorraine H. Kligman[a], *Elaine Schwartz*[b], *Robert H. Lesnik*[a], *James A. Mezick*[c]

Departments of Dermatology,
[a] University of Pennsylvania, School of Medicine, Philadelphia, Pa., and
[b] Mt. Sinai School of Medicine, New York, N.Y.;
[c] R.W. Johnson Pharmaceutical Research Institute, Raritan, N.J., USA

Prolonged topical use of potent corticosteroids results in the well-known atrophic features that include skin thinning, increased transparency and telangiectasia [1, 2]. The marked thinning has been produced in both animal and human skin. Contributory factors include a reduction in epidermal thickness [3, 4] and a profound reduction in dermal glycosaminoglycans leading to collapse of the three-dimensional array of collagen bundles [5]. The loss of glycosaminoglycans and proteoglycans has been confirmed in animals biochemically [6, 7]. In vivo and in vitro studies report inhibition of collagen synthesis [8–10].

Even more well-known are the significant beneficial effects of corticosteroids in many inflammatory diseases. Because of their value and extensive use, it would be desirable to increase the benefit/risk ratio of these drugs. For a number of reasons, we believed that retinoids would have the ability to do so. Many of the activities of retinoids run counter to those of steroids. For example, instead of being atrophogenic, they induce epidermal hyperplasia [11, 12]. Retinoids have been shown to stimulate collagen synthesis in the repair of photodamaged connective tissue [13, 14], in normal wound healing [15] and in steroid-inhibited wound healing [16]. In addition, there is increasing evidence that retinoids may have mild anti-inflammatory activity [17, 18].

To explore our hypothesis, we examined the ability of tretinoin (all-*trans*-retinoic acid) to inhibit steroid atrophy in mice by in vivo, histological [19] and biochemical means. The lack of interference with the anti-inflammatory property of steroids was assessed in two model systems.

Materials and Methods

Animals
In all experiments but one, mice were 8-week-old Skh-hairless-1 females (Skin and Cancer Hospital, Temple University Health Sciences Center, Philadelphia, Pa., USA). In the ear edema experiment, CD/1 albino haired mice were used. Mice were housed individually with free access to food and water.

Steroids
For studies of histological atrophy and skin inflammation the following steroids were used: 0.05% clobetasol propionate cream, 0.1% halcinonide cream, 0.05% betamethasone valerate cream, 0.025% fluocinolone acetonide (FA) cream and, in ethanol, 0.05% FA and 0.1% triamcinolone acetonide.

The in vivo skin-fold thickness test utilized dexamethasone (DEX) in alcohol/propylene glycol (70:30 v/v) at 3 concentrations (0.1, 0.05 and 0.01%). Ear edema studies also used DEX in the same vehicle but at 1.0, 0.1 and 0.01% concentrations. The steroid used for the biochemical studies was 0.05% clobetasol propionate in an ethanol/propylene glycol vehicle (70:30 v/v).

Assessment of Skin Atrophy
Histology. Two treatment regimens were adopted: (1) steroid creams (clobetasol propionate, halcinonide, betamethasone valerate) in the morning with tretinoin cream (0.025 or 0.05%) in the afternoon, 5 days a week for 3 weeks, and (2) steroids in ethanol (FA, triamcinolone acetonide) with tretinoin in ethanol (0.025 and 0.1%) applied immediately after each steroid treatment for 14 consecutive days. Appropriate vehicle controls were included. Each treatment group contained 4 mice. Dorsal skin biopsy specimens were processed for light microscopy and stained with hematoxylin and eosin.

Skin-Fold Thickness. Six to 8 mice were treated dorsally with 100 µl of DEX at the 3 concentrations in the morning and either vehicle or 0.025% tretinoin cream in the afternoon for 9 consecutive week days. Appropriate controls were included. Topical agents were prepared each day. Twenty-four hours after the final treatment, double skin-fold thickness was measured with an electronic digital caliper (model MAX-CAL, Cole-Parmer, Chicago, Ill., USA) with an accuracy of ± 0.03 mm.

Assessment of Anti-Inflammatory Effects
Ear Edema Model. The dorsal surface of the left ears of two large groups of CD/1 mice was pretreated either with 20 µl of 0.025% tretinoin or the acetone vehicle. The right ears served as untreated controls. One hour later, the left ears (10 mice per group) were treated either with 0.05% 12-O-tetradecanoylphorbol-13-acetate (TPA) in acetone or 0.05% TPA and DEX at 3 concentrations. Appropriate controls were included. Five and a half hours

after the final treatment, 7-mm punch biopsy specimens were taken from both ears and weighed on an electric balance. The difference between the treated and untreated ears of the same animal was the measure of edema.

Skin Inflammation Model. The dorsal trunk skin (9 mice per group) was treated with 0.5% croton oil in mineral oil, in the morning. Treatment in the afternoon was either with FA cream alone, FA cream and 0.0125% tretinoin cream, or nothing for 5 days. On days 6–10 only the afternoon treatments were performed. Three mice per group were sacrificed on the morning of days 6, 9 and 11. Dorsal skin biopsy specimens were processed for light microscopy with hematoxylin-eosin stain.

Biochemistry Studies. Three groups of 20 hairless mice each, aged 6–8 weeks, were treated topically for 3 weeks on a morning:afternoon schedule as follows: (1) vehicle:vehicle; (2) steroid:vehicle, and (3) steroid:tretinoin [0.05% in the ethanol/propylene glycol (70:30 v/v) vehicle]. Applications were 100 μl to the dorsal trunk. Mice were sacrificed on the day after the final treatment. Dorsal trunk skin was frozen for quantification of glycosaminoglycans and fibronectin.

Glycosaminoglycan Analysis. Skins were defatted and suspended in 0.1 M phosphate buffer (pH 6.5) with 0.005 M EDTA and 0.005 M cysteine HCl. Digestion with papain was for 24 h at 65 °C. After centrifugation, the supernatant was diluted with water and the glycosaminoglycans precipitated with cetylpyridinium chloride. The precipitate was dissolved in *n*-propanol and further precipitated with absolute ethanol and a few drops of saturated sodium acetate. The glycosaminoglycans were dissolved in water, transferred to preweighed tubes and dried, after which the glycosaminoglycan weight was calculated. Glycosaminoglycans were redissolved in water and uronic acid content was determined by the carbazole assay [20].

Fibronectin Analysis. Skins were trimmed to equal surface area, homogenized, defatted and extracted with 0.05 M Tris HCl (pH 7.5), 1.0% sodium dodecyl sulfate, 0.33 M mercaptoethanol and proteolytic inhibitors. The supernatants were electrophoretically concentrated and analyzed for fibronectin content by a specific ELISA utilizing rabbit antimouse fibronectin and purified mouse fibronectin.

Results

Assessment of Skin Atrophy

Histology. Atrophy was produced by all steroids tested. The normal epidermis of 3–4 cell layers was thinned to 2 layers, the cells of which were condensed with scanty cytoplasm. The dermis was thin as was the subcutaneous panniculus carnosus. Frequent tearing during sectioning suggested fragility (fig. 1a).

In both treatment regimens, whether tretinoin was applied several hours after the steroid or immediately after, it prevented the corticosteroid-induced atrophy (fig. 1b). Epidermis was thickened with 6–8 layers, the cells of which had abundant cytoplasm. A prominent granular layer, typical for tretinoin treatment, was usually present. The dermis contained densely deposited collagen bundles and the panniculus carnosus was of normal dimensions.

Table 1. Skin-fold thickness: dose response

Treatment		n	Double skin-fold thickness, mm (mean ± SE)
morning	afternoon		
Vehicle	Vehicle	8	0.934 ± 0.086
0.1% DEX	Vehicle	6	0.587 ± 0.035*
0.05% DEX	Vehicle	8	0.725 ± 0.038*
0.01% DEX	Vehicle	8	0.911 ± 0.052
0.1% DEX	0.025% RA	7	0.837 ± 0.075
0.05% DEX	0.025% RA	6	0.917 ± 0.091
0.01% DEX	0.025% RA	8	0.933 ± 0.103
0.025% RA	Vehicle	8	1.059 ± 0.112

DEX = Dexamethasone; RA = all-*trans*-retinoic acid (tretinoin).

* $p < 0.05$ versus vehicle control (Dunnett's two-tailed t test). Reprinted from Lesnik et al. [19] with permission from Mosby, St. Louis, Mo., USA.

Skin-Fold Thickness. A significant dose-dependent thinning was produced by 0.1 and 0.05% DEX compared to vehicle controls ($p < 0.05$). Tretinoin, applied in the afternoon, prevented the thinning (table 1). Application of tretinoin alone thickened the skin slightly, compared to the vehicle control, but the difference was not significant.

Assessment of Anti-Inflammation

Ear Edema. TPA-induced ear edema was reduced in a dose-dependent manner by DEX. The addition of tretinoin to DEX had no effect on the inhibition (fig. 2). The concentration of DEX required to reduce ear edema by 50% (ED_{50}) was similar with and without tretinoin (0.056 and 0.052%, respectively), showing that DEX and DEX plus tretinoin were equipotent. Neither tretinoin alone nor vehicle had an effect on the edema.

Skin Inflammation. A robust epidermal hyperplasia (8–10 cell layers) was produced by 5 days' application of croton oil. This was accompanied by a severe dermal inflammatory infiltrate consisting of many lymphocytes, fewer eosinophils and still fewer neutrophils. Vessels were dilated and engorged with red blood

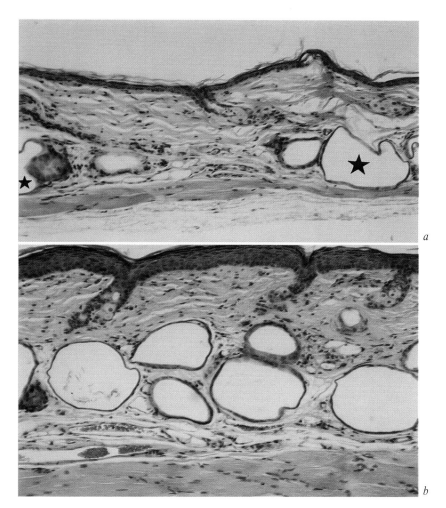

Fig. 1. a Atrophy induced by betamethasone valerate (0.05%) is characterized by thinning of the epidermis, dermis and subcutaneous muscle layer. Tearing of the collagen matrix and partial collapse of the dermal cysts (star), a normal feature of the hairless mouse, was typically seen. Hematoxylin-eosin stain. ×95. *b* Tretinoin (0.05%) applied after betamethasone valerate (0.05%) prevented the atrophic changes. The epidermis is hyperplastic and dermal components are restored to normal dimensions and architecture. Hematoxylineosin. ×95. [From ref. 19, with permission from Mosby.]

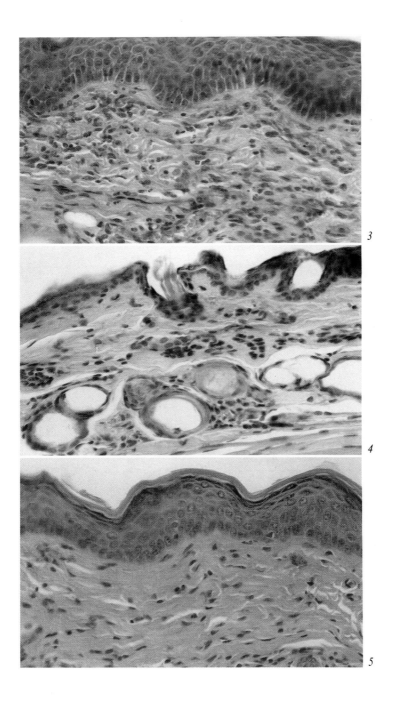

3

4

5

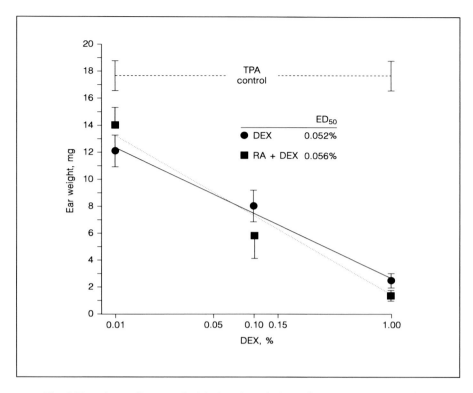

Fig. 2. Ear edema. Compared with the edema induced in TPA controls, application of either DEX alone or DEX and tretinoin (all-*trans*-retinoic acid; RA) reduces the edema in an equivalent and dose-related manner. ED_{50} = Reduction of ear edema by 50%. [From ref. 19, with permission from Mosby.]

Fig. 3. Croton oil (0.05%): 5 days application. Biopsy specimen taken 5 days later. A severe inflammatory infiltrate along with engorged blood vessels is present. The epidermis is very hyperplastic with intercellular edema. Hematoxylin-eosin stain. × 200. [From ref. 19, with permission from Mosby.]

Fig. 4. Croton oil (0.05%) for 5 days followed by FA (0.025%) for 5 days. Dermal inflammation is greatly reduced with residual cellularity consisting mainly of atrophic follicular epithelial cells. The epidermis and dermis are atrophic. Hematoxylin-eosin stain. × 200. [From ref. 19, with permission from Mosby.]

Fig. 5. Croton oil (0.5%) for 5 days followed by FA (0.025%) and tretinoin (0.01%) for 5 days. Inflammation is greatly reduced with residual dermal cellularity consisting mainly of fibroblasts. The epidermis is orderly and hyperplastic without edematous changes and the granular layer is prominent. Hematoxylin-eosin stain. × 200. [From ref. 19, with permission from Mosby.]

cells. These features were still present, with only slight amelioration, 5 days after the croton oil applications were stopped (fig. 3).

Application of FA after each croton oil treatment and then for another 5 days greatly reduced inflammation and vascular dilation. However, the epidermis was atrophic (2–3 cell layers) with condensed basophilic cells (fig. 4). The collagen-containing upper dermis was also thinned.

When FA and tretinoin were applied, inflammation was reduced as with FA alone (fig. 5). Dermal cellularity was still elevated but this was due to fibroplasia. Notably, both epidermal and dermal atrophy were prevented.

Similar results were obtained when all three agents were applied for only 5 days.

Biochemical Analysis. Glycosaminoglycans were decreased by the steroid treatment and were stimulated to higher than normal levels when steroid was followed by tretinoin. This was evident by all means of measurement (table 2).

Steroid treatment increased the fibronectin content of the skin, compared to controls. When followed by tretinoin, the steroid-elevated fibronectin content was substantially reduced, bringing it closer to normal values (table 3).

Discussion

An active area of pharmaceutical research is focussed on the production of steroids that exert their anti-inflammatory effect without causing atrophy. Whether or not this goal is fully achieved remains to be seen. In the meantime, this study does provide evidence that the atrophogenic and anti-inflammatory properties of steroids can be dissociated. We have shown that tretinoin can counteract the undesirable effect yet leave the beneficial capability intact.

Because of the multifarious effects of retinoids on skin [11–13, 21–23], the mechanisms underlying the abrogation of atrophy are also likely to be numerous. Prevention of epidermal thinning may result from the ability of tretinoin to induce DNA synthesis [17], followed by hyperplasia of epidermal cells [11, 12].

Prevention of dermal atrophy probably involves many components. Steroid inhibition of collagen synthesis is well documented [8–10, 24, 25]. While the brief treatment times in these studies would appear insufficient to affect such a stable molecule as collagen, Young et al. [6] reported a decrease in the hydroxyproline content of rat skin after only 11 applications of 0.01% triamcinolone acetonide. Equally as rapid is the retinoid stimulation of collagen synthesis. Ehrlich et al. [26] found significantly more collagen in sponges implanted in rats at days 3 and 7 after treatment with both steroid and vitamin A than was found in controls treated with the steroid alone. In control rats, treated only with vitamin A, a small increase in collagen was found at day 7.

Table 2. Quantification of glycosaminoglycans

Treatment	Cetylpyridinium chloride precipitation			Uronic acid content		
	$\mu g/mg$ w.w.	$\mu g/mg$ d.w.	$\mu g/cm^2$	$\mu g/mg$ w.w.	$\mu g/mg$ d.w.	$\mu g/cm^2$
Vehicle:vehicle	5.57	23.65	193	0.22	0.94	7.66
Steroid:vehicle	3.67	17.88	108	0.15	0.73	4.39
Steroid:tretinoin	7.03	26.98	237	0.37	1.43	12.57

w.w. = Wet weight; d.w. = dry weight.

Table 3. Fibronectin content

Treatment group	Fibronectin content		
	ng/mg w.w.	ng/mg d.w.	ng/cm^2
Vehicle:vehicle (I)	1.68 ± 0.10	7.83 ± 0.50	79.0 ± 14.4
Steroid:vehicle (II)	3.55 ± 0.26	14.45 ± 1.03	114.5 ± 10.2
Steroid:tretinoin (III)	2.71 ± 0.35	10.23 ± 1.13	107.7 ± 6.25
Statistical analysis I vs. II	$p < 0.001$	$p < 0.001$	$p < 0.05$
(Student's t test) I vs. III	$p < 0.01$	$p < 0.05$	$p < 0.05$
II vs. III	$p < 0.05$	$p < 0.012$	n.s.

w.w. = Wet weight; d.w. = dry weight.

The tretinoin-induced increases in proteoglycans and glycosaminoglycans are probably a major factor in the prevention of dermal atrophy. The rapid depletion of these macromolecules by steroids has been described by Lehmann et al. [5] in humans and by Särnstrand et al. [7] in rats. Histologically, this is difficult to perceive in hairless mice because of the normal paucity of this material [27]. Retinoids have been shown to enhance the production of glycosaminoglycans in vitro [28, 29]. In this study we confirm, biochemically, that in vivo glycosaminoglycans are significantly decreased by even short-term steroid treatment and that tretinoin not only prevents their depletion, but raises them to higher than normal levels.

The role of fibronectin in dermal atrophy is less clear. It has been reported to be diminished by steroids [30]. On the other hand, more recent studies report higher than normal levels of fibronectin after in vitro addition of steroids [31–33]. Our studies are in agreement with the latter work showing a 2-fold increase in the fibronectin content of steroid-treated mouse skin. Tretinoin reduced the increase but levels remained higher than in normal controls. This may reflect the reported ability of retinoids themselves to increase fibronectin [29] and may be yet another example of the modulating property of retinoids whereby they have different effects in normal and abnormal tissue. Other examples are the retinoid-induced decrease in epidermal proliferation in psoriasis [34] versus its stimulation in normal epidermis [11] and the suppression of collagen synthesis in keloid fibroblasts [35] versus its increased deposition in normal dermis [36].

The mechanism behind the retinoid noninterference with steroid anti-inflammatory behavior is not understood. It could be just that: noninterference. However, the putative anti-inflammatory property of retinoids [17] may play a role. In addition, the often reported retinoid enhancement of the immune system [37–39] may stimulate anti-inflammation processes that have not yet been elucidated.

The potential for atrophy, whether from topical or systemic steroids [40], is a serious drawback. The elimination of this major side effect with topical tretinoin would have significant clinical implications as it increases the benefit/risk ratio for steroid therapy.

References

1   Schöpf E: Side effects from topical corticosteroid therapy. Ann Clin Res 1975;7:353–367.
2   Stevanovic DV: Corticosteroid-induced atrophy of the skin with telangiectasia. A clinical and experimental study. Br J Dermatol 1972;87:548–566.
3   Winter GD, Burton JL: Experimentally induced steroid atrophy in the domestic pig and man. Br J Dermatol 1976;94(suppl 12):107–109.
4   Kirby JD, Munro DD: Steroid-induced atrophy in an animal and human model. Br J Dermatol 1976;94(suppl 12):111–119.
5   Lehmann P, Zheng P, Lavker RM, Kligman AM: Corticosteroid atrophy in human skin: A study by light, scanning and transmission electron microscopy. J Invest Dermatol 1983;81:169–176.
6   Young JM, Yoxall BE, Wagner BM: Corticosteroid-induced dermal atrophy in the rat. J Invest Dermatol 1977;69:458–462.
7   Särnstrand B, Brattsand R, Malmström A, Kobayasi T: Effects of glucocorticoids on dermal proteoglycans. J Invest Dermatol 1983;80:340.
8   Uitto J, Teir H, Mustakallio KK: Corticosteroid-induced inhibition of the biosynthesis of human skin collagen. Biochem Pharmacol 1972;21:2161–2167.
9   McCoy BJ, Diegelmann RE, Cohen IK: In vitro inhibition of cell growth, collagen synthesis and prolyl hydroxylase activity by triamcinolone acetonide. Proc Soc Exp Biol Med 1980;163:216–222.
10 Sterling KM Jr, Harris MJ, Mitchell JJ, Di Petrillo TA, Delaney GL, Cutroneo KR: Dexamethasone decreases the amounts of type I pro-collagen mRNAs in vivo and in fibroblast cell cultures. J Biol Chem 1983;258:7644–7647.

11 Connor MJ, Lowe NJ, Ashton RE: Retinoids induce epidermal proliferation at sub-toxic doses. J Invest Dermatol 1984;82:431a.

12 Elias PM: Epidermal effects of retinoids: Supramolecular observations and clinical implications. J Am Acad Dermatol 1986;15:797–809.

13 Kligman LH, Chen HD, Kligman AM: Topical retinoic acid enhances the repair of ultraviolet-damaged dermal connective tissue. Connect Tissue Res 1984;12:139–150.

14 Schwartz E, Cruickshank FA, Mezick JA, Kligman LH: Topical all-trans retinoic acid stimulates collagen synthesis in vivo. J Invest Dermatol 1991;96:975–978.

15 Lee KH, Tong TG: Mechanism of action of retinyl compounds on wound healing. II. Effect of active retinyl derivatives on granuloma formation. J Pharm Sci 1970;59:1195–1197.

16 Hunt TK, Ehrlich HP, Garcia JA, Dunphy JE: Effect of vitamin A on reversing the inhibitory effect of cortisone on healing of open wounds in animals and man. Ann Surg 1969;170:633–641.

17 Hensby CN, Eustache J, Shroot B, Bouclier M, Chatelus A, Luginbuhl B: Anti-inflammatory aspects of systemic and topically applied retinoids. Agents Actions 1987;21:238–240.

18 Tsambaos D, Orfanos CE: Effects of oral retinoid on dermal components of human and animal skin; in Orfanos CE, Braun-Falco O, Farber EM, Grupper C, Polano MK, Schuppli R (eds): Retinoids: Advances in Basic Research and Therapy. Berlin, Springer, 1981, pp 99–108.

19 Lesnik RH, Mezick JA; Capetola R, Kligman LH: Topical all-trans-retinoic acid prevents corticosteroid-induced skin atrophy without abrogating the anti-inflammatory effect. J Am Acad Dermatol 1989;21:186–190.

20 Bitter T, Muir HM: A modified uronic acid carbazol reaction. Anal Biochem 1962;4:330–334.

21 Fisher GJ, Esmann J, Griffiths CEM, Talwar HS, Duell EA, Hammerberg C, Elder JT, Karabin GD, Nickoloff BJ, Cooper KD, Voorhees JJ: Cellular, immunologic and biochemical characterization of topical retinoic acid-treated human skin. J Invest Dermatol 1991;96:699–707.

22 Fisher GJ, Tavakkol A, Griffiths CEM, Elder JT, Zhang Q-Y, Finkel L, Danielpour D, Glick AB, Higley H, Ellengsworth L, Voorhees JJ: Differential modulation of transforming growth factor-$\beta1$ expression and mucin deposition by retinoic acid and sodium lauryl sulfate in human skin. J Invest Dermatol 1992;98:102–108.

23 Elder JT, Fisher GJ, Zhang Q-Y, Eisen D, Krust A, Kastner P, Chambon P, Voorhees JJ: Retinoic acid receptor gene expression in human skin. J Invest Dermatol 1991;96:425–433.

24 Ponec M, Kempenaar JA, Van der Meulen-Van Harskamp GA, Bachra BN: Effects of glucocorticosteroids on cultured human skin fibroblasts. IV. Specific decrease in the synthesis of collagen, but no effect on its hydroxylation. Biochem Pharmacol 1979;28:2777–2783.

25 Shull S, Cutroneo KR: Glucocorticoids coordinately regulate procollagens type I and III synthesis. J Biol Chem 1983;258:3364–3369.

26 Ehrlich HP, Tarver H, Hunt TK: Effects of vitamin A and glucocorticoids upon inflammation and collagen synthesis. Ann Surg 1973;177:222–227.

27 Kligman LH, Akin FJ, Kligman AM: Prevention of ultraviolet damage to the dermis of hairless mice by sunscreens. J Invest Dermatol 1982;78:181–189.

28 Shapiro SS, Poon JP: Effect of retinyl acetate on sulfated glycosaminoglycan biosynthesis in dermal and epidermal cells in vitro. Connect Tissue Res 1978;6:101–108.

29 Roberts AB, Sporn MB: Cellular biology and biochemistry of the retinoids; in Sporn MB, Roberts AB, Goodman DS (eds): The Retinoids. Orlando, Academic Press, 1984, vol 2, pp 210–286.

30 Fyrand O: Studies on fibronectins in the skin. VIII. Influence of corticosteroids on cell cultures from normal human skin. Acta Derm Venereol (Stockh) 1985;65:379–384.

31 Babu M, Diegelmann R, Oliver N: Fibronectin is overproduced by keloid fibroblasts during abnormal wound healing. Mol Cell Biol 1989;9:1642–1650.

32 Russel SB, Trupin JS, Myers JC, Broquist AH, Smith JC, Myles ME, Russell JD: Differential glucocorticoid regulation of mRNAs in human dermal fibroblasts: Keloid-derived and fetal fibroblasts are refractory to down-regulation. J Biol Chem 1989;264:13730–13735.

33 Nimmer D, Bergstrom G, Hirano H, Amrani DL: Regulation of plasma fibronectin by glucocorticoids in chick hepatocyte cultures. J Biol Chem 1987;262:10369–10375.

34 Frost P, Weinstein GD: Topical administration of vitamin A acid for ichthyosiform dermatoses and psoriasis. JAMA 1969;207:1863–1868.
35 Abergel RP, Meeker CA, Oikarinen H, Oikarinen AI, Uitto J: Retinoid modulation of connective tissue metabolism in keloid fibroblast cultures. Arch Dermatol 1985;121:632–635.
36 Kligman LH, Mezick JA, Capetola RJ, Thorne EG: Lifetime topical application of tretinoin to hairless mice. Acta Derm Venereol (Stockh) 1992, in press.
37 Lin T-H, Chu TM: Enhancement of murine lymphokine-activated killer cell activity by retinoic acid. Cancer Res 1990;50:3013–3018.
38 Sidell N, Ramsdell F: Retinoic acid upregulates interleukin 2-receptors on activated human thymocytes. Cell Immunol 1988;115:299–309.
39 Valone FH, Payan DG: Potentiation of mitogen-induced human T-lymphocyte activation by retinoic acid. Cancer Res 1985;45:4128–4131.
40 de Lacharrière O, Escoffier C, Teillac D, Saint-Leger D, Debure A, Leveque JL, Kreiss H, de Prost Y: Reversal effects of systemic corticotherapy by topical tretinin in grafted kidney patients. Pharmacol Skin 1989;3:51–60.

Lorraine H. Kligman, PhD, University of Pennsylvania, School of Medicine,
Rm. 227, Clinical Research Bldg., 422 Curie Blvd., Philadelphia, PA 19104 (USA)

Korting HC, Maibach HI (eds): Topical Glucocorticoids with Increased Benefit/Risk Ratio.
Curr Probl Dermatol. Basel, Karger, 1993, vol 21, pp 89–96

....

Ranking of Topical Glucocorticoids

Principles and Results

Eric W. Smith, John M. Haigh

School of Pharmaceutical Sciences, Rhodes University, Grahamstown, South Africa

The increasing synthesis and use of topical corticosteroid products over the past 30 years has necessitated the development of suitable methods for evaluating the efficacy and potency of new drug entities. Several in vivo models have been developed in this regard using laboratory animals and human subjects (table 1). Generally, these tests measure the difference in the non-immunological inflammatory response to an exogenous inflammatory mediator in the presence and absence of the corticosteroid under test. There are also immunologically based assays and several tests which assess the antiproliferative effects of the drug. Several comparative disease model evaluations have also been developed using human subjects. Most of these assays are non-ideal from one point of view or another: most are invasive methods which require some form of trauma to be induced in the skin and therefore problematic to perform and monitor.

In comparison, the human skin blanching assay for topical corticosteroids is relatively simple to perform and does not require any trauma on the part of the volunteers. This assay makes use of the skin whitening (blanching) side effect of topical corticosteroid application, the intensity of the blanching correlating directly with the drug potency or success of drug delivery through the stratum corneum [1, 2]. The blanching intensity has also been shown to correlate directly to the clinical efficacy of the preparation [3, 4]. In addition the blanching assay may be conducted in a relatively short time (2 days), thereby eliminating the lengthy assessment period of other in vivo assays. The first documented use of the blanching (or vasoconstriction) assay by McKenzie and Stoughton appeared in 1962 [5], although the use of the skin whitening effect of hydrocortisone on

Table 1. In vivo methods used to assess topical corticosteroid efficacy and potency

Animal models	Human models
Non-immunological inflammation models	Non-immunological inflammation models
Croton oil erythema test	Croton oil–kerosene erythema test
Cantharidin test	Ultraviolet-induced erythema test
Ultraviolet-induced erythema test	Pyrogen erythema test
Immunological inflammation models	Disease models
Hypersensitivity tests	Psoriasis plaque assay
Assessment of antimitotic effects	Poison ivy test
Hyperplasia models	Assessment of adverse effects
Atrophy models	Atrophy tests
Wound healing models	Ammonium hydroxide blister test
	Stratum corneum thickness tests
	Acne tests
	Tests for systemic effects

stripped skin was reported by Wells in 1957 [6]. The exact mechanism by which the skin whitening is generated remains unclear, hence the preferred name of blanching rather than vasoconstriction assay [7].

Assay Methodology

The optimized methodology [2] of the skin blanching assay utilizes 12–15 fair-skinned volunteers who are proven responders to topical corticoid application; a small percentage of the population do not demonstrate the blanching side-effect to these drugs (although still respond clinically in the normal way). Full disclosure of information regarding the assay and acquisition of informed consent is practised in the normal way. The subjectivity of the methodology requires 3 independent, trained observers to be used for valid data recording. Investigation has shown that participation in 3 trials provides sufficient experience for a novice observer to become sufficiently skilled in discerning different intensities of skin blanching [8]. The subjectivity of the assay also requires a rigorous double-blind coding protocol to prevent any bias on the part of the observers. The corticoid products to be evaluated are usually coded by a third party not involved in the trial. Four random application patterns are drawn up each comprising 12 application sites. The products to be compared are randomly assigned to these sites so that each formulation is represented an equal number of times and, importantly, applied along the entire length of the forearm [9]. Each arm of each volunteer is randomly assigned 1 of the 4 patterns.

Twelve discrete application sites are demarcated on each arm of each volunteer by the application of 6 self-adhesive labels that have had two 7×7 mm squares punched from their centres. Each square represents one application site and is numbered in a standard manner. The products to be tested are either extruded from a small syringe which has had the needle cut to a length of approximately 5 mm; four 7-mm 'stripes' of formulation extruded in this way approximate 3 mg of formulation [10]. Alternatively, 3 μl of liquid formulation may be applied to each site using a micropipette. After application the formulations are uniformly spread over the entire application site using a glass rod. Once all the sites have been filled, one arm of each volunteer is occluded by covering each site with water-impervious tape, the other arm has its sites guarded using a perspex frame which does not prevent evaporation from the skin or formulation but does prevent accidental abrasion. In this manner both the clinical application modes of occlusion and non-occlusion may be tested. The formulations, tapes and dressings remain on the skin for 6 h after which they are removed and any residual formulation is washed from the skin with water and the arm patted dry. Any erythema or skin puckering from the tape usually subsides within 30 min after removal. The first observation of skin blanching is made 1 h after product removal (7 h after application).

The blanching response is independently assessed by the 3 observers on 10 occasions between 7 and 32 h after corticosteroid application. The intensity of skin whitening is subjectively graded on a 0–4 scale, 0 representing no blanching, 4 representing intense blanching with distinct margins, and 1, 2 and 3 representing the intermediate grades. After the final observation the score sheets are decoded and the scores summated for generation of a blanching profile and statistical analysis. The blanching profile is plotted as response in the form of percentage of total possible score (%TPS) versus time. The TPS is the product of the maximum score per site, the number of observers, the number of sites per arm for each preparation and the number of volunteers. The actual score (AS) is the sum of the frequencies for each grade recorded. The %TPS is the quotient of AS and TPS multiplied by 100. The blanching profiles generated in this way allow normal topical availability comparisons as well as estimations of peak blanching, time to peak and duration of blanching.

In an attempt to assess the precision of this assay methodology, we have conducted a retrospective analysis of all the trials conducted in our laboratories over the last 20 years. We usually include Betnovate cream as a standard formulation into every trial conducted. If the profile obtained for Betnovate has the usual characteristic shape then the credence of the other results is strengthened. The results of several thousand observations in this manner show good precision in both the occluded and unoccluded modes of application [11].

Results

This blanching assay methodology may be used for a number of different comparative evaluations: one use has been the screening of new drug molecules for clinical activity [12–17]. When used for this purpose the different characteristic blanching response profiles of betamethasone 17-valerate and fluocinolone acetonide, for example, are evident: the latter has a slower onset, higher peak response and longer duration than the former [18]. This is also a good example for illustrating the misleading results that may be obtained by single-point observation protocols. Any single observation between 0 and 12 h, where the blanching responses are approximately equal, would suggest equivalence between these two formulations, only full-curve monitoring will demonstrate the superiority of fluocinolone acetonide.

The blanching assay has been used extensively for potency ranking of corticoid formulations [19–21]. Eumovate (clobetasone butyrate) has been compared to Betnovate and Dermovate in our laboratories [22] and demonstrates the moderate potency of the test formulation when compared to these standards. Interestingly, Eumovate ointment induces higher blanching in the unoccluded application mode compared to the occluded mode, an unexplained phenomenon which is not observed with any other formulations. The blanching assay has also been used for determining optimal application regimens for topical formulations [23].

The blanching assay may be used for comparing topical availability of the same drug from the same type of delivery vehicle [24–28]; comparative topical availability assessments of this type are routinely conducted for regulatory purposes. It is obvious from these studies that the corticosteroid may be delivered to the stratum corneum in very different amounts from two formulations of the same type (creams for example) which both contain the same drug in the same concentration, but differ in the other formulation excipients [18].

The human skin blanching assay may also provide interesting results that influence the clinical choice of drug delivery vehicle. Markedly different topical availabilities of the same corticosteroid are often observed when comparing drug delivery from different formulation types (creams, ointments, gels and solutions) containing the same concentration of drug [29, 30]. One would assume that different vehicles of the same label concentration would deliver similar quantities of drug to the skin. Our experience shows that alcoholic solutions allow much more drug to penetrate the skin than do ointments or oil-in-water creams and lotions. Occlusion greatly enhances drug availability from lotion formulations, but has relatively little effect on the ointment formulation. This is important clinically because these relatively potent lotion and alcoholic solution vehicles are usually applied to the face and scalp, skin which is inherently more permeable than that of many other anatomical regions.

The assay may also be usefully applied to the assessment of penetration enhancer effects on topical corticosteroid availability [31–33]. The effects of penetration enhancers such as oleic acid or propylene glycol may be assessed using the human skin blanching assay. The blanching response results depicted in figure 1 indicate the effect of adding these penetration enhancers to an extemporaneous formulation containing betamethasone 17-valerate. In the case of these results the commercial formulation (Betnovate cream) generated the least blanching in both the occluded and unoccluded application test modes. Even the extemporaneous control formulation which contained neither propylene glycol nor oleic acid performed better than the commercial formulation. The presence of

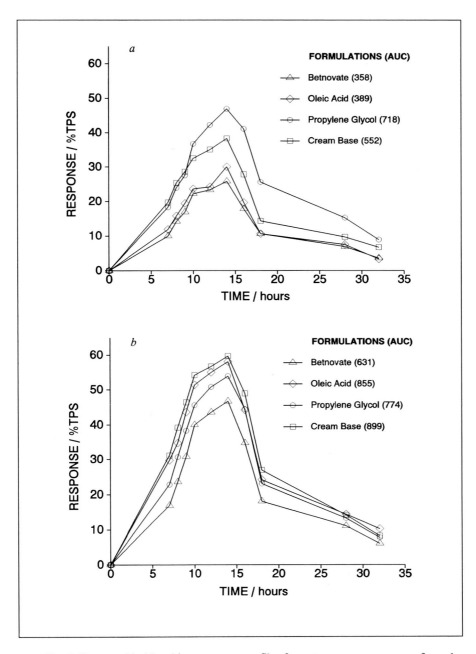

Fig. 1. Human skin blanching response profiles for extemporaneous cream formulations containing penetration enhancers and commercial Betnovate cream. *a* Unoccluded application mode. *b* Occluded application mode.

propylene glycol in the formulation generated some improvement in drug release compared to the control formulation in the unoccluded application mode; however, neither penetration enhancer demonstrated superiority to the control cream in the occluded mode.

It is interesting to note that a common result observed in our laboratories is repeated in these results: we have almost exclusively found that extemporaneous test formulations perform better than commercial products when compared by the human blanching assay. Furthermore, we have compounded micronized formulations that contain one tenth the drug concentration of commercial products but still elicit greater response profiles due to optimized delivery vehicle microstructure [34]. It must be stressed that long-term stability studies have not been conducted on these extemporaneous formulations and hence we cannot comment on the shelf lives of these products compared to the commercial formulations. However, it seems clear that we should be able to improve the rate and extent of drug delivery by optimizing the chemical and physical composition of the topical vehicle, when compared to products that are already on the market. Such an optimization should have marked clinical, toxicological and financial implications.

Conclusions

Although relatively crude in methodology, the skin blanching assay remains an accurate, reproducible and rapid method of assessing topical corticosteroid availability and potency. There has lately been criticism of the subjectivity of the assay and suggestions that optical methods may yield more 'meaningful' results [7, 35]. On reviewing the literature one finds that numerous instrumental techniques have been evaluated over the last 2 decades as potential alternatives to the visual assessment of the skin whitening response. These techniques have all demonstrated inferior or equivalent results compared to visual methodology. However, being cumbersome and time-consuming, none of these instrumental methods has replaced visual assessment procedures as a routine practice. As research advances with newer optical instruments [36], the replacement of the current subjective assessment may certainly be justified.

Acknowledgements

The financial assistance from Rhodes University Council, the Foundation for Research Development and Cassella-Riedel Pharma GmbH is acknowledged with gratitude.

References

1   Haigh JM, Kanfer I: Assessment of topical corticosteroid preparations: The human skin blanching assay. Int J Pharm 1984;19:245–262.
2   Smith EW, Meyer E, Haigh JM, Maibach HI: The human skin blanching assay as an indicator of topical corticosteroid bioavailability and potency: An update; in Bronaugh RL, Maibach HI (eds): Percutaneous Absorption. Mechanisms – Methodology – Drug Delivery, 2nd ed, New York, Dekker, 1989, pp 443–460.
3   Cornell RC, Stoughton RB: Correlation of the vasoconstriction assay and clinical activity in psoriasis. Arch Dermatol 1985;121:63–67.
4   Barry BW, Woodford R: Activity and bioavailability of topical steroids: In vivo/in vitro correlations for the vasoconstrictor test. J Clin Pharmacol 1978;3;43–65.
5   McKenzie AW, Stoughton RB: Method for comparing percutaneous absorption of steroids. Arch Dermatol 1962;86:608–610.
6   Wells GC: The effect of hydrocortisone on standardized skin-surface trauma. Br J Dermatol 1957; 69:11–18.
7   Haigh JM, Smith EW: Topical corticosteroid-induced skin blanching measurement: Eye or instrument? Arch Dermatol 1991;127:1065.
8   Smith EW, Meyer E, Haigh JM: The human skin blanching assay for topical corticosteroid bioavailability assessment; in Shah V, Maibach HI (eds): Cutaneous Bioavailability, Bioequivalence and Penetration. New York, Plenum, in press.
9   Meyer E, Smith EW, Haigh JM: Sensitivity of different areas of the flexor aspect of the human forearm to corticosteroid-induced skin blanching. Br J Dermatol 1992;127:379–381.
10   Magnus AD, Haigh JM, Kanfer I: Assessment of some variables affecting the blanching activity of betamethasone 17-valerate cream. Dermatologica 1980;160:321–327.
11   Smith EW, Meyer E, Haigh JM: Accuracy and reproducibility of the multiple-reading skin blanching assay; in Maibach HI, Surber C (eds): Topical Corticosteroids. Basel, Karger, 1992, pp 65–73.
12   Baker H, Sattar HA: The assessment of four new fluocortolone analogues by a modified vasoconstriction assay. Br J Dermatol 1968;80:46–53.
13   Bluefarb SM, Howard FM, Liebsohn EI, Schlagel CA, Wexler L: Diflorasone diacetate: Vasoconstrictor activity and clinical efficacy of a new topical corticosteroid. J Int Med Res 1976;4:454–461.
14   Druzgala P, Hochhaus G, Bodor N: Soft drugs. 10. Blanching activity and receptor binding affinity of a new type of glucocorticoid–loteprednol etabonate. J Steroid Biochem Mol Biol 1991;38:149–154.
15   Grubstad E, Bengtsson B: A comparison of a new steroid, budesonide, with other topical corticosteroids in the vasoconstriction assay. Drugs Exp Clin Res 1980;6:385–390.
16   Ishihara M: Studies on the vasoconstrictor activity of amcinonide: A new synthetic topical corticosteroid. Nishi-Nihon Hitu 1976;38:285–293.
17   Woodford R, Barry BW: Activity and bioavailability of a new steroid (timobesone acetate) in cream and ointment compared with Lidex and Dermovate creams and ointments and Betnovate cream. Int J Pharm 1985;26:145–155.
18   Smith EW, Meyer E, Haigh JM, Maibach HI: The human skin blanching assay for comparing topical corticosteroid availability. J Dermatol Treatm 1991;2:69–72.
19   Poulsen BJ, Burdick K, Bessler S: Paired comparison vasoconstrictor assays: A comparison of methods for the determination of relative vasoconstrictor potency of topically applied corticosteroids. Arch Dermatol 1974;109:367–371.
20   Schalla W, Schorning S: Potency assessment of topical corticoids in the vasoconstrictor assay and on tuberculin-induced inflammation. Skin Pharmacol 1991;4:191–204.
21   Poulsen J, Rorsman H: Ranking of glucocorticoid creams and ointments. Arch Dermatol 1980;60: 57–62.
22   Meyer E, Smith EW, Haigh JM, Kanfer I: Potency ranking of two new topical corticosteroid creams containing 0.1% desonide or 0.05% halometasone utilising the human skin blanching assay. Drug Res 1988;38:1840–1843.

23 Woodford R, Haigh JM, Barry BW: Possible dosage regimens for topical steroids, assessed by vaso-constrictor assays using multiple applications. Dermatologica 1983;166:136–140.

24 Barry BW, Woodford R: Comparative bio-availability of proprietary topical corticosteroid prepa-rations: Vasoconstrictor assays on thirty creams and gels. Br J Dermatol 1974;91:323–338.

25 Barry BW, Woodford R: Comparative bio-availability and activity of proprietary topical corticoste-roid preparations: Vasoconstrictor assays on thirty-one ointments. Br J Dermatol 1975;93:563–571.

26 Barry BW, Woodford R: Propriety hydrocortisone creams: Vasoconstrictor activities and bio-avail-abilities of six preparations. Br J Dermatol 1976;95:423–425.

27 Meyer E, Haigh JM, Kanfer I: Comparative bioavailability of some locally manufactured betame-thasone valerate containing preparations. S Afr Pharm J 1983;50:445–447.

28 Meyer E, Kanfer I, Haigh JM: Comparative blanching activities of some topical corticosteroid containing lotions. S Afr Pharm J 1981;48:551–552.

29 Woodford R, Barry BW: Bioavailability and activity of betamethasone 17-benzoate in gel and cream formulations: Comparison with proprietary topical corticosteroid preparations in the vaso-constrictor assay. Curr Ther Res 1974;16:338–343.

30 Smith EW, Meyer E, Haigh JM: Blanching activities of betamethasone formulations: The effect of dosage form on topical drug availability. Drug Res 1990;40:618–621.

31 Bennett SL, Barry BW, Woodford R: The assessment of some potential penetration enhancers using the vasoconstrictor test. J Pharm Pharmacol 1984;36:8P.

32 Barry BW, Southwell D, Woodford R: Optimization of bioavailability of topical steroids: Penetra-tion enhancers under occlusion. J Invest Dermatol 1984;82:49–52.

33 Woodford R, Barry BW: Alphaderm cream (1% hydrocortisone plus 10% urea): Investigation of vasoconstrictor activity, bioavailability and application regimens in human volunteers. Curr Ther Res 1984;35:759–767.

34 Haigh JM, Smith EW, Meyer E, Fassihi R: Influence of the oil phase dispersion in a cream base on the in vivo release of betamethasone 17-valerate. STP Pharma Sci 1992;2:259–264.

35 Shah VP, Peck CC, Skelly JP: Vasoconstriction – Skin blanching-assay for glucocorticoids: A cri-tique. Arch Dermatol 1989;125:1558–1561.

36 Chan SY, Li Wan Po A: Quantitative skin blanching assay of corticosteroid creams using tristimu-lus colour analysis. J Pharm Pharmacol 1992;44:371–378.

Eric W. Smith, PhD, School of Pharmaceutical Sciences, Rhodes University,
PO Box 94, Grahamstown 6140 (South Africa)

Korting HC, Maibach HI (eds): Topical Glucocorticoids with Increased Benefit/Risk Ratio.
Curr Probl Dermatol. Basel, Karger, 1993, vol 21, pp 97–106

······························

Suppression of Induced Inflammation in Man

M.J. Kerscher

Department of Dermatology, Ludwig Maximilian University, Munich, FRG

Topical glucocorticoids are still among the most frequently used dermatics. This is due to their undebatable potency in inflammatory skin diseases. Their therapeutic efficacy in a wide spectrum of dermatoses depends predominantly on their anti-inflammatory activity (AIA) [1]. The second main effect is their antimitotic activity which is needed in diseases with increased cell turnover and seems to be linked with skin atrophy, the most serious unwanted effect of topical glucocorticoids [2]. Besides skin atrophy, a suppression of the hypothalamic-pituitary-adrenal axis is mostly feared [3, 4]. Much effort is taken to reduce these events. Besides the alteration of the steroid nucleus to modify drug binding to the steroid receptors, more recently research has focused on a change in the structural aspects determining the mode of delivery to obtain high drug concentrations in the target tissue [5, 6]. Pertinent steroids include halogenated ones (mometasone furoate) and the nonhalogenated double esters [7–9].

Among these soft steroids as they are sometimes called, there are two different groups, first the prednisone-derived substances like prednicarbate and 6-methylprednisolone aceponate, and second the hydrocortisone-derived substances like hydrocortisone aceponate and hydrocortisone buteprate. Previous experience with these steroids has shown a lack of atrophogenicity in normal human skin as assessed by high-frequency ultrasound [10, 11]. Moreover, some clinical trials addressing the above-mentioned glucocorticoids indicate that the efficacy of prednicarbate, hydrocortisone aceponate and hydrocortisone buteprate is in the order of magnitude of that of betamethasone 17-valerate [12–14].

There is, however, a lack of studies conforming to present standards in clinical pharmacology which demonstrate the efficacy and safety of these nonhalogenated double esters. This holds true both with respect to the effects in experimental dermatoses induced in healthy volunteers and the efficacy in various inflammatory skin diseases, e.g. atopic eczema. In particular, the AIA of the nonhalogenated double esters has not yet been compared. The same holds true with respect to the influence of the vehicle and – even more – the drug concentration. These, however, are important parameters.

In the present study we compared in healthy volunteers using two assay systems the AIA of 3 or 5 prednicarbate preparations to that of cream preparations with two other nonhalogenated double esters, betamethasone 17-valerate and hydrocortisone 1%, as well as 2 base preparations.

Methods

Design

These were two double-blind randomized studies. The AIA was assessed using the ultraviolet B (UVB)-induced erythema test and the vasoconstriction assay of McKenzie and Stoughton [15].

After approval by the local ethical committee, 42 healthy volunteers were included in the study after having given written informed consent. They had no history of skin disease and no hypersensitivity to glucocorticoids or ingredients of topical dermatics/cosmetics, presented no intense sun tanning of the test area, and took no glucocorticoids systemically or topically on large surface areas during 6 weeks or any drug treatment on the test area for at least 7 days prior to the study. The test area was the skin of the upper back of either side of the vertebral column. Blood samples for blood count, serum creatinine, aspartate aminotransferase, alanine aminotransferase and γ-glutamyltransferase were taken at the beginning and at the end of the study.

Test Preparations

The following test preparations were used in the first part of the study (UVB-induced erythema test): (1) prednicarbate 0.25% cream (Dermatop® Creme); (2) prednicarbate 0.1% cream; (3) prednicarbate 0.05% cream; (4) corresponding vehicle to preparations 1–3; (5) betamethasone 17-valerate 0.1% cream; (6) hydrocortisone 1.0% cream; (7) hydrocortisone aceponate 0.1% cream; (8) hydrocortisone buteprate 0.1% cream, and (9) base cream DAC (unguentum emulsificans aquosum; Deutscher Arzneimittel Codex).

Test preparations used in the second part of the study (vasoconstriction assay) were: (1) prednicarbate cream 0.5% (50% water); (2) prednicarbate cream 0.25% (50% water); (3) prednicarbate 0.25% (Dermatop® Creme); (4) prednicarbate 0.1% cream; (5) prednicarbate 0.05% cream; (6) prednicarbate 0.025% cream; (7) corresponding vehicle to preparations 3–6; (8) betamethasone 17-valerate 0.1% cream; (9) hydrocortisone 1.0% cream; (10) hydrocortisone aceponate 0.12% cream; (11) hydrocortisone buteprate 0.1% cream, and (12) base cream DAC.

The test preparations were kept in neutral, coded syringes.

UV-Induced Erythema Test

In the first part of the study an erythema induced by UVB light was used as assay to study the AIA of the above-mentioned test preparations. 18 healthy volunteers (8 males/10 females with an age range from 22 to 36 years and a mean age of 29.6 years) were recruited.

Table 1. Study design of the UVB-induced erythema test

	Day 1	Day 2	Day 3
Light step (for the MED)	×		
Visual determination of MED		×	
Irradiation (2 MEDs)		×	
Visual score			×
Chromametry			×

MED = Minimal erythema dose.

The study design has already been described [16–18] and is demonstrated in table 1. After determination of the minimal erythema dose by a stepwise increase in UVB doses, the test areas, first marked with a water-resistant pen, were irradiated with 2 minimal erythema doses. Untested skin was protected. Immediately after irradiation 0.2 ml of the test preparations was applied to one of the 10 test areas following the random plan. One area remained untreated and served for control. After application of the test preparations the treatment sites were covered nonocclusively with cotton gauze and fixed with Leukosilk® plaster to ensure skin contact. 23 h thereafter the cotton gauze was removed, and 1 h later each site was assessed for degree of erythema by subjective assessment and by objective measurements with a chromameter.

The observer, a study-blind person, inspected test sites visually using a score (0 = no effect; 1 = slight reduction of erythema, 2 = marked, but not absolute suppression of erythema, 3 = no erythema) for the determination of the degree of erythema.

For the objective assessment of erythema, a Minolta chromameter CR 200 (Minolta, Ahrensburg, FRG), consisting of a reflected light colorimeter with 6 silicon photocells, was used. The changes in skin redness (Δa^*) and total skin color (ΔE^*) as compared to an untreated area of the back served for analysis.

Vasoconstriction Test

The second part of the study was the investigation of the blanching effects of the different glucocorticoid preparations following a study design first described by McKenzie and Stoughton [15] and then modified by Haigh and Kanfer [19] as well as by Smith et al. [20]. The assay procedure employed 24 healthy volunteers (9 males/15 females with an age range from 23 to 39 years and a mean age of 30.5 years). Exclusion criteria were the same as mentioned above.

12 areas (2 × 3 cm) were demarcated with a water-resistant pen. Uniform amounts of the different glucocorticoid formulations to be evaluated were applied to these sites by extrusion from a 1-ml syringe following the random plan. The extruded formulations were spread over the application sites using glass rods. One area remained again untreated and served for control. The preparations were coded prior to application to maintain the double-blind nature of this investigation. In the first 12 volunteers the application sites were covered with Oclufol® (Lohmann, Neuwied, FRG), a polyethylene film which prevented the evaporation of moisture and the delivery of vehicle components. In the other 12 volunteers

the application sites remained unoccluded, but they were covered with cotton gauze which should prevent accidental removal of the applied formulations by abrasion. The test preparations remained in contact with the skin for 6 h. After this time the cotton gauze or the occlusive dressing were carefully removed. Residual formulation was gently removed from the application sites. 1 h later 2 observers assessed the degree of induced blanching on each site at regular intervals. Observations were made at 7, 8, 10, 12, 24, 32 and 48 h after the initial application. The degree of blanching was determined by subjective assignment of a number between 0 and 3 representing the perceived intensity of blanching at each site (0 = normal skin; 3 = intensive, absolute blanching). Furthermore, the degree of blanching was assessed with a Minolta chromameter as described above.

Side Effects

The test areas were inspected at each visit for adverse effects and the subjects were asked for adverse events.

Statistics

This is an explorative study. The sums of the individual score values (sum scores) and mean values of Δa^* and ΔE^* are given. Skin redness or blanching following the application of the various test preparations were related to one another and the control area by the Wilcoxon-Pratt test. Moreover, in the vasoconstriction assay, the AUC values were calculated by standard trapezoidal summation. Thus, a topical availability curve was produced for each preparation and allowed comparative examination of the preparations tested. $p <$ 0.05 was considered to indicate a difference.

Results

UV-Induced Erythema Test

UV irradiation induced marked erythema at 24 h. As described earlier in more detail [21], the various preparations markedly influenced UVB-induced erythema (table 2, fig. 1). The highest reduction of erythema as compared to the control area was obtained by hydrocortisone buteprate. When comparing the sum scores of the different prednicarbate formulations as assessed in the UVB erythema test, prednicarbate 0.25% proves more potent than prednicarbate 0.1% and prednicarbate 0.05% (table 3). These data give evidence for a clear dose-response relationship of prednicarbate in the UVB-induced erythema test.

Vasoconstriction Test

There are some striking differences between the occlusive and the nonocclusive part of the vasoconstriction assay (fig. 2, 3) [21]. Table 4 gives the mean values of the visual score for the entire observation period of the occlusive part of the vasoconstriction assay. Statistical analysis (AUC values) suggests prednicarbate 0.1% as well as prednicarbate 0.5% to be superior to prednicarbate 0.25%. There are no statistically significant differences between betamethasone 17-valerate and

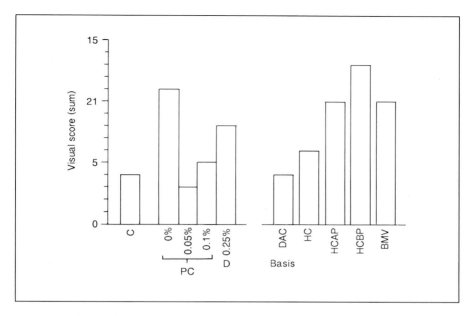

Fig. 1. Sums of the visual scores (UV erythema test, nonocclusive) in 18 volunteers 24 h after irradiation with 2 minimal erythema doses and application of the test preparations: C = control; PC = prednicarbate; D = Dermatop® 0.25% (prednicarbate); DAC = unguentum emulsificans aquosum (Deutscher Arzneimittel Codex); HC = hydrocortisone; HCAP = hydrocortisone aceponate; HCBP = hydrocortisone buteprate; BMV = betamethasone 17-valerate. [From 21, with permission.]

Table 2. Sums of the visual scores (UV-induced erythema test, nonocclusive) in 18 volunteers 24 h after irradiation with 2 minimal erythema doses and application of the test preparations

Preparation	Sum score
Prednicarbate 0.05%	3
Base cream DAC	4
Prednicarbate 0.1%	5
Hydrocortisone	6
Dermatop 0.25%	8
Betamethasone 17-valerate/hydrocortisone aceponate	10
Hydrocortisone buteprate	13

Suppression of Induced Inflammation in Man

Table 3. Sum scores of the different prednicarbate formulations according to the UVB-induced erythema test

Preparation	Sum score
Prednicarbate 0.05%	3
Prednicarbate 0.1%	5
Dermatop 0.25%	8

Table 4. Mean values of the sum scores in 12 volunteers over the entire observation period of the vasoconstriction assay (occlusive part)

	Mean visual score after 12 h
Prednicarbate 0.1%	1.06
Prednicarbate 0.5%	0.95
Hydrocortisone aceponate	0.90
Hydrocortisone buteprate	0.86
Dermatop 0.25%	0.69
Betamethasone 17-valerate	0.60
Prednicarbate 0.025%	0.55
Prednicarbate 0.25%	0.38
Prednicarbate 0.05%	0.33
Prednicarbate 0%	0.14
Hydrocortisone	0.12
Base cream DAC	0.06

Fig. 2. AUC values in the occlusive part of the vasoconstriction assay (12 volunteers) shown as columns (= upper and lower quartile of median; large star = median; encircled star indicates a difference to prednicarbate 0.25% (p < 0.05); small star = values outside the upper and lower quartile of median. PC = Prednicarbate; D = Dermatop® 0.25%; L = lipophilic vehicle containing 0.25 or 0.5% prednicarbate; DAC = unguentum emulsificans aquosum (DAC); HCAP = hydrocortisone aceponate; HCBP = hydrocortisone buteprate; BMV = betamethasone 17-valerate. [From 21, with permission.]

Fig. 3. AUC values in the nonocclusive part of the vasoconstriction assay (12 volunteers). For explanation of the symbols, see legend to figure 2.

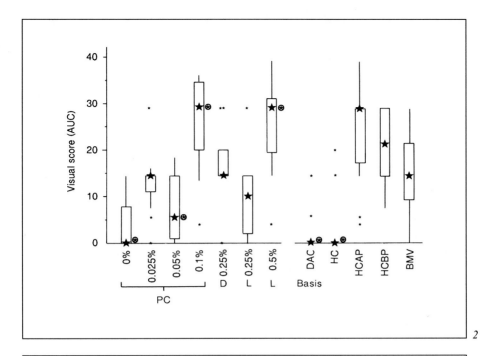

2

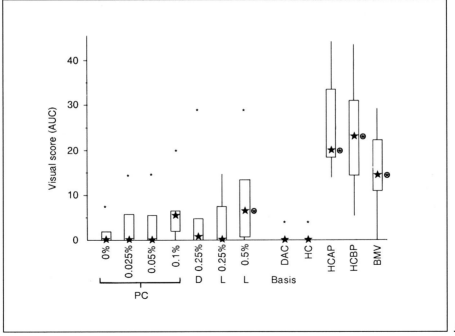

3

the nonfluorinated double esters prednicarbate, hydrocortisone aceponate and hydrocortisone buteprate in the occlusive part of the vasoconstriction assay.

The results of the nonocclusive part of the vasoconstriction assay are shown in figure 3. Statistical analysis (AUC values) suggests prednicarbate 0.1% as well as 0.5%, hydrocortisone buteprate, hydrocortisone aceponate and betamethasone 17-valerate to be superior to prednicarbate 0.25%.

Drug- as well as vehicle-related side effects were not observed or reported by the subjects taking part in the UV erythema test and the vasoconstriction assay [21].

Discussion

A variety of methods have been proposed for the measurement of the AIA of topical glucocorticoids [22]. We have assessed the AIA of newly developed topical glucocorticoids of the nonfluorinated double ester type and conventional medium-potent and weak glucocorticoids using two models of inflammation: the UVB-induced erythema test, a relatively new model of inflammation, as well as the vasoconstriction assay of McKenzie and Stoughton [15], a classical test for assaying the AIA of topical glucocorticoids.

Subjective and objective parameters served for analysis. In general, chromametry turned out to be less discriminatory as compared to visual inspection. This fact has already been described by Wilhelm et al. [23]. The suppression of skin redness induced by UV irradiation was most pronounced following hydrocortisone buteprate. Visual scoring demonstrated also a remarkable AIA of hydrocortisone aceponate, betamethasone 17-valerate and prednicarbate 0.25%. This is well in accordance with clinical trials in eczema which indicated a comparable antiphlogistic effect of prednicarbate and betamethasone 17-valerate [13]. As expected, prednicarbate 0.05% and 0.1% appeared less active.

The skin blanching effect induced by the occlusive application of the various topical glucocorticoids was most pronounced following the application of prednicarbate 0.1% and 0.5% which induced more skin blanching than prednicarbate 0.25%. This result, however, needs definite proof.

A remarkable skin blanching effect was also induced by prednicarbate 0.25%, hydrocortisone aceponate and hydrocortisone buteprate which are altogether glucocorticoids of the nonhalogenated double ester type. Because of their high AIA, their reduced skin-atrophogenic potential and their high clinical efficacy, these newly developed glucocorticoids may have an increased benefit/risk ratio.

The results of the nonocclusive part of the vasoconstriction assay were striking. In this part of the study, hydrocortisone aceponate, hydrocortisone buteprate, betamethasone 17-valerate and prednicarbate 0.5% (lipophilic vehicle) were clearly more potent than prednicarbate 0.25%, which was about as active as prednicarbate 0.05%, 0.025% and 0.1%, incorporated in a hydrophilic vehicle. One reason for the different result may be the incidental removal or uptake of the applied preparation by the cotton gauze. Another reason for this result may be that there is a higher delivery and bioavailability of the glucocorticoid from the vehicle containing 78% water when applied occlusively. This should be analyzed further.

In conclusion, the present study demonstrates a high AIA of all nonhalogenated double esters tested. Given that their clinical efficacy is in the order of magnitude of that of betamethasone 17-valerate and that their atrophogenic potential is in the order of magnitude of that of vehicle preparations, these new glucocorticoid formulations may have an increased benefit/risk ratio.

This should be proven in a clinical trial comparing the efficacy of the above-mentioned glucocorticoids with that of medium-potent conventional glucocorticoids by use of objective and subjective techniques, e.g. defined visual scores as well as high-frequency ultrasound, profilometry, chromametry and transepidermal water loss. The possibility to perform such trials in reality is, however, limited, as the comparison of various congeners of a certain type of a glucocorticoid is almost excluded.

Acknowledgment

The tables and figures in this article are taken or modified from [21] with permission.

References

1   Robertson DB, Maibach HI: Topical corticosteroids. Int J Dermatol 1982;21:59–67.
2   Akers WA: Risks of unoccluded topical steroids in clinical trials. Arch Dermatol 1980;116:786–788.
3   Scoggins RB, Kligman B: Percutaneous absorption of corticosteroids: Systemic effects. N Engl J Med 1965;273:831–840.
4   Gell KA, Baxter DL: Plasma cortisol depression by steroid creams. Arch Dermatol 1964;89:734–740.
5   Töpert M: Perspectives in corticosteroid research. Drugs 1988;36(suppl 5):1–8.
6   Thalen A, Brattsand R, Andersson PH: Development of glucocorticosteroids with enhanced ratio between topical and systemic effects. Acta Derm Venereol (Stockh) 1989;69(suppl 151):11–19.
7   Medansky RS, Bressinck R, Cole GW, et al: Mometasone furoate ointment and cream 0.1 percent in treatment of psoriasis: Comparison with ointment and cream formulations of fluocinolone acetonide 0.025 percent and triamcinolone acetonide 0.1 percent. Cutis 1988;42:480–485.
8   Katz HI, Prawer SE, Watson MJ, Scull TA, Peets EA: Mometasone furoate ointment 0.1% vs. hydrocortisone ointment 1.0% in psoriasis. Int J Dermatol 1989;28:342–344.

9   Bodor N: The application of soft drug approaches to the design of safer corticosteroids; in Christophers E, et al (eds): Topical Corticosteroid Therapy: A Novel Approach to Safer Drugs. New York, Raven Press, 1988, pp 13–25.

10 Korting HC, Vieluf D, Kerscher M: 0.25% prednicarbate cream and the corresponding vehicle induce less skin atrophy than 0.1% betamethasone 17 valerate cream and 0.05% clobetasol propionate. Eur J Clin Pharmacol 1992;42:159–161.

11 Kerscher MJ, Korting HC: Topical glucocorticoids of the non-fluorinated double ester type: Lack of atrophogenicity in normal human skin as assessed by high frequency ultrasound. Acta Derm Venereol (Stockh) 1992;72:214–216.

12 Flasch CI, Klaschka F: Therapeutisches Profil des ersten Hydrocortisondiesters in lipophiler Grundlage. Dtsch Dermatol 1986;7:806–828.

13 Vogt HJ, Höhler Th: Controlled studies of intraindividual and interindividual design for comparing corticoids clinically; in Christophers E, et al (eds): Topical Corticosteroid Therapy: A Novel Approach to Safer Drugs. New York, Raven Press, 1988, pp 169–180.

14 Hevert F, Schipp I, Busch B, Rozman T: Kortikosteroid-Ester. Dtsch Dermatol 1989;10:678–683.

15 McKenzie AW, Stoughton RB: Method for comparing the percutaneous absorption of steroids. Arch Dermatol 1962;86:608–610.

16 Ljunggren B, Möller H: Influence of corticosteroids on ultraviolet light erythema and pigmentation in man. Arch Dermatol Forsch 1973;248:1–12.

17 Kerscher MJ: Influence of liposomal encapsulation on the activity of a herbal non-steroidal antiinflammatory drug; in Braun-Falco O, Korting HC, Maibach HI (eds): Liposome Dermatics. Berlin, Springer, 1992, pp 329–337

18 Korting HC, Schäfer-Korting M, Hart H, Laux P, Schmid M: Antiinflammatory activity of Hamamelis distillate applied topically to the skin. Influence of vehicle and dose. Eur J Clin Pharmacol 1993;44:315–318.

19 Haigh JM, Kanfer I: Assessment of topical corticosteroid preparations: The human skin blanching assay. Int J Pharmacol 1984;19:245–262.

20 Smith EW, Meyer E, Haigh JM, Maibach HI: The human skin blanching assay for comparing topical corticosteroid availability. J Dermatol Treatm 1991;2:69–72.

21 Schäfer-Korting M, Korting HC, Kerscher MJ, Lenhard S: Prednicarbate activity and benefit/risk ratio in relation to other topical glucocorticoids. Clin Pharmacol Ther, in press.

22 Wendt H, Frosch PJ: Klinisch-pharmakologische Modelle zur Prüfung von Corticoidexterna. Basel, Karger, 1982.

23 Wilhelm KP, Surber C, Maibach HI: Quantification of sodium lauryl sulfate irritant dermatitis in man: Comparison of four techniques: Skin colour reflectance, transepidermal water loss, laser Doppler flow measurement and visual scores. Arch Dermatol Res 1989;281:293–295.

Dr. M.J. Kerscher, Dermatologische Klinik und Poliklinik der Ludwig-Maximilians-Universität, Frauenlobstrasse 9–11, D–80337 München (FRG)

Korting HC, Maibach HI (eds): Topical Glucocorticoids with Increased Benefit/Risk Ratio.
Curr Probl Dermatol. Basel, Karger, 1993, vol 21, pp 107–113

....

The Psoriasis Plaque Test and Topical Corticosteroids: Evaluation by Computerized Laser Profilometry

H.H. Wolff, J.F. Kreusch, K.-P. Wilhelm, S. Klaus

Department of Dermatology, Medical University of Lübeck, FRG

Numerous methods are available for the determination of general effects, especially the therapeutic efficacy of topical corticosteroids [1, 2], for example, the blanching test; pyrexal erythema test; epicutaneous patch test; ammonium hydroxide blister test; Duhring chamber test for teleangiectasia; corticoid horny layer test; ultrasound assessment of atrophogeneity; psoriasis plaque test, and contact dermatitis suppression test.

An important one is the well-established psoriasis plaque test which evaluates effects of local application of corticosteroids onto a chronic psoriatic lesion. In contrast, most other models require the induction of an 'artificial' inflammatory skin lesion and subsequent local therapy. Testing the efficacy of topical corticosteroids in psoriasis may be of greater relevance for practical application of steroid preparations [3–5]. However, most of the tests are difficult to evaluate quantitatively. We report a possible improvement of the evaluation of the psoriasis plaque test.

Psoriasis Plaque Test

For this test, long-standing plaques of psoriasis are treated with various samples of topical corticosteroid preparations and appropriate controls. The test areas are evaluated at standardized time intervals by visual/sensual determination of: erythema (0–3 points), scaling (0–3 points), and infiltrate (0–3 points). Addition of the points leads to a final score ranging from 0 to 9 [4].

It is obvious that this visual evaluation even if performed by two independent investigators is rather an estimate than an exact measurement. Especially for comparison of preparations with only slightly differing therapeutic strengths, a more precise method would be desirable.

Various instrumental measuring techniques have therefore been applied, for example: skin color reflectance measurement; laser Doppler flowmetry; determination of transepidermal water loss (TEWL), and profilometry.

Methods determining parameters of blood perfusion of the skin (color reflectance, blood flow) or water loss through the epidermis are quite sensitive, but the measurements may easily be disturbed by climatic and other environmental factors as well as by the status of the proband. It is well known that blushing and transpiration of a person may be influenced by nutritional (alcohol!) and emotional factors.

Thus it may be advantageous not to measure parameters depending on skin perfusion or water loss (functional/dynamic parameters), but to use morphological parameters which are rather independent of the current status of the patient and the environment. It is a clinical experience that the roughness of a psoriatic lesion decreases under therapy. Various methods (image analysis, optical interferometry, scanning electron microscopy, profilometry, etc.) have been proposed to determine 'roughness' of the skin [6–10]. In the past, profilometry was performed with instruments using a stylus for tracking profile altitudes of the skin [11, 12]. The introduction of computerized laser profilometers permits an expanded, rapid and detailed analysis of structures of the skin surface, including determination of roughness and other parameters. The function of these profilometers will be explained below. The laser profilometer yields more information than instruments using a stylus.

Computerized Laser Profilometry

The application of industrial laser profilometers to dermatological measuring problems has been developed in our department using a UBM instrument (UBC 14 central unit, UBM Microfocus laser sensor, UBM Messtechnik GmbH, Ettlingen, FRG). The principle of this technique is illustrated in figure 1: The beam (b) of a semiconductor laser source (a, wavelength 780 nm) is focused by means of a motile lens (c) onto the surface of a silicone skin replica to give a spot of 1 µm in diameter (d). The traversing table (e) carrying the replica is moved in a meander-like fashion by two computer-controlled precision motors providing defined movement in the x- and y-direction. Up to 1,000 points/mm may be scanned. The laser beam reflected from the surface of the replica is projected onto photodiodes (g) via a prism (f). Any defocusing of the beam due to peaks or

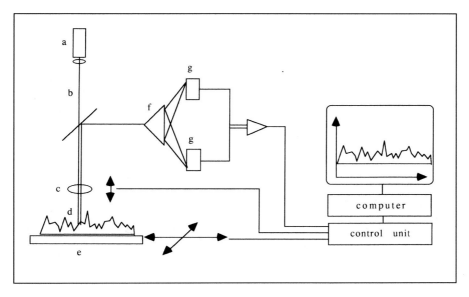

Fig. 1. Schematic drawing of the computerized laser profilometry system.

furrows of the replica is registered by the diodes, which causes the computer to move the lens until new focusing is achieved. During the scanning procedure the position of the lens is registered digitally by the computer, the value represents the information of the height at the particular position of the replica. As a result of the x,y-controlled movement of the traversing table the whole area of a specimen may be scanned. Figure 2 shows the original setup of the measuring system. As the scanning of a surface requires several minutes, the system cannot be used for direct measurements on living skin. The use of silicone replicas has been proven to represent very precisely the surface of the skin. Systematic testing of various silicone impression materials has given the best results for Silflo (Flexico, J.&S. Davis, Potters Bar, Herts., UK) with regards to our measuring problems. Figure 3 shows the taking of a replica [13].

Practical Applications of Computerized Laser Profilometry

The technique can be used for: (a) reconstruction of the three-dimensional surface of a skin specimen (from a silicone replica); (b) calculation of the roughness parameters according to industrial standards (DIN, ISO), and (c) analysis of surface structures by mathematical procedures (Fourier transform, power spectra).

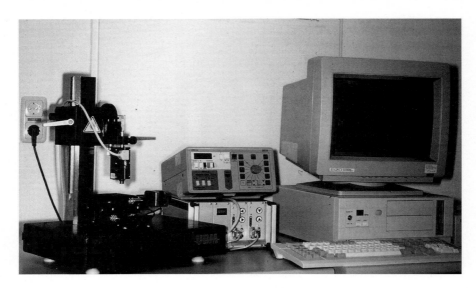

Fig. 2. Setup of the measuring system. Left: Traversing table and laser source; center: control unit; right: computer and screen.

Reconstruction of the Three-Dimensional Surface of the Skin

From the data recorded concerning the position of the lens and of the x,y-table, a three-dimensional reconstruction of the surface of the skin is created on the computer screen. Height intervals may be coded by different colors. Thus the image contains visible information about the peaks and grooves of the normal or diseased skin surface. Figure 3a–c demonstrates as an example psoriatic skin prior to (fig. 3a) and after 16 days of treatment (fig. 3b) with anthralin. Though clinically at this time the skin appeared already normal, the comparison to normal skin of the same patient (fig. 3c) revealed still considerable irregularities and height differences of the treated area.

Calculation of Roughness Parameters

The calculation of roughness parameters from the original data is only possible after elimination of superimposed elements of form and waviness of the original profiles by mathematical procedures [14]. This has been done with the data

Fig. 3. Three-dimensional reconstruction of the surface of a psoriatic plaque before (*a*) and after (*b*) treatment with anthralin, in comparison to normal skin of the same patient (*c*).

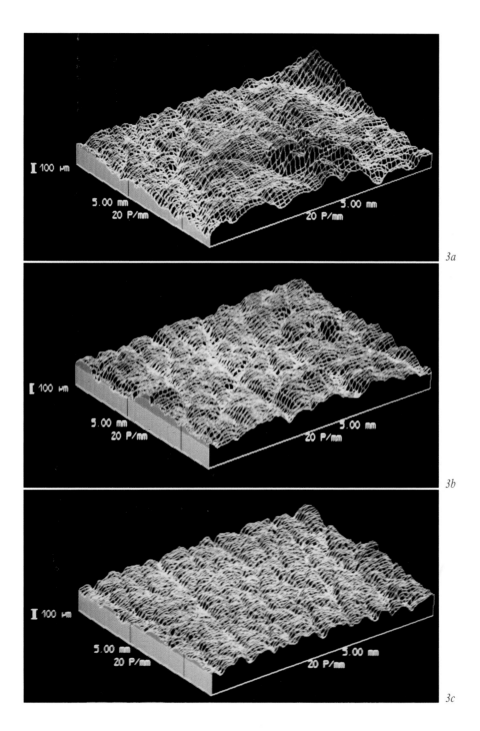

3a

3b

3c

Psoriasis Plaque Test Evaluation by Computerized Laser Profilometry   Plate I

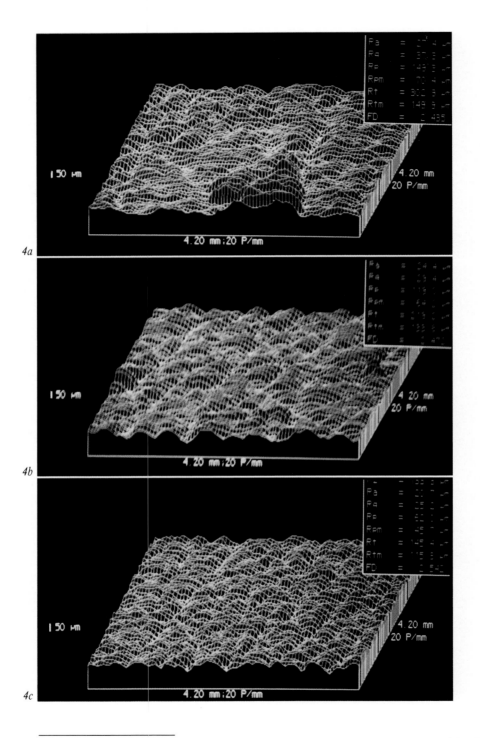

4a

4b

4c

from the examples of figure 3a–c, resulting in figure 4a–c. The calculation of roughness parameters covering the whole area is achieved according to industrial standards (DIN, ISO). In our example various parameters (R_z, R_a) clearly decline over the time of treatment. However, there remains still a difference to the values of normal skin (fig. 4c). This underlines the advantage of exact measurements over the 'clinical impression'.

Analysis of the Surface Structures and Profiles

The profiles of the surface of the skin are composed of periodical (regular) and stochastic (irregular) elements. By means of a Fourier transform, the frequencies of the complex wave patterns may be analyzed.

The autocorrelation function separates periodical and stochastic elements of the profiles and thus evaluates the regularity (periodicity) of the structures. Power spectra represent the direction and amplitudes of regular waves over the area.

The application of these procedures is demonstrated in the following example: In the course of a psoriasis plaque test, prednicarbate ointment was compared to an indifferent base preparation serving as control. Clinically, after 7 days of treatment, the psoriatic test field had completely cleared (fig. 5a, b). Reconstruction of the relief showed change from irregularity (fig. 5c) to regularity (fig. 5d), as well as the decrease of the calculated roughness parameters. The autocorrelation function revealed almost complete lack of periodic structures in the psoriatic field prior to treatment, the central peak of figure 5e represents the stochastic components of the profiles. After treatment (fig. 5f), apart from the stochastic elements (center), the periodic structures reappeared, which are typical of normal skin. The power spectra demonstrate the presence of waves of low frequency and high amplitude before treatment (center of the plot, fig. 5g). After treatment (fig. 5h), waves of higher frequency and lower amplitude appeared. This is typical of normal skin. The area treated with a base preparation showed only slight decreases in roughness parameters, as an effect of the occlusion. However, autocorrelation function and power spectra remained unchanged. This example underlines that not the schematic, unreflected consideration of roughness parameters may be most important, but the mathematical analysis of surface patterns. The clearing of a psoriatic lesion is not only characterized by the change of the surface from 'rough' to 'smooth', but also from 'chaos' to 'order'.

Fig. 4. Roughness profiles and calculated roughness parameters of a psoriatic plaque before (a, R_z 280.4 µm, R_a 27.4 µm) and after (b, R_z 178.1 µm, R_a 24.4 µm) treatment with anthralin, in comparison to normal skin of the same patient (c, R_z 133.3 µm, R_a 20.7 µm).

Comparison of Laser Profilometry to Other Methods

Although laser profilometry is more time-consuming than for example measurements of skin color reflectance or TEWL, the method yields results which reflect the clinical appearance of healthy and diseased skin. Roughness and smoothness are parameters not only important in following the course of skin diseases, but also for estimating effects of cosmetic products on normal skin. Obviously measurement of erythema, for example, is not helpful for the latter problem. Certainly determination of dynamic parameters is advantageous for other questions. Although the necessity for taking replicas includes the possibility of making technical mistakes, usually the silicone rubber prints are of high precision and give stable reproductions of the surface of the skin. Morphology of the surface is less subject to deviations of environmental factors and physical condition of the patient at the moment of taking the replica than dynamic parameters. One of the major advantages of laser profilometry is the use of an optical instrument instead of a mechanical stylus. The laser beam may be focused to smaller diameters (1 µm) than the radius of the tip of the stylus (5 µm). Thus a more precise recording of very fine details of the surface is possible without mechanical alteration of the probe. In mechanical instruments the stylus is usually mounted to a sledge which is drawn across the area to be scanned. Stylus and sledge may cause mechanical alterations of the very sharp crests of the replica which represent the fine furrows of the skin in a negative cast. An optical instrument does not cause any mechanical damage to the surface of the probe and permits repeated measurements. Due to the computerized recording of the data the whole area is scanned with the laser profilometer, whereas some stylus instruments just record 12 radial tracks at 30° intervals each. The laser instrument yields information covering the whole area and due to the sharply focused beam and the very fine step intervals of the x,y-motors, even very small areas may be scanned precisely. If appropriately small steps are selected for scanning, the reconstruction on the computer screen yields images almost as detailed as photographs. Rapid evaluation of the data is achieved using powerful hardware to make best use of the program supplied by the manufacturer. Various roughness parameters may be calculated by the program. The analysis of the wave pattern of the profiles has become quite simple and first results are promising as to obtaining important information of biologic relevance concerning regularity of the skin surface analyzed. Work is going on to evaluate which parameters correlate best with the clinical impression

Fig. 5. Psoriasis plaque test with prednicarbate ointment: Clinical image prior to (*a*) and after 7 days of treatment (*b*). Reconstruction of the surface profiles and calculation of roughness parameters before (*c*, R_z 285.0 µm, R_a 35.9 µm) and after treatment (*d*, R_z 194.5 µm, R_a 23.7 µm). Autocorrelation function (*e, f*) and power spectra (*g, h*) are calculated for the corresponding intervals (see text).

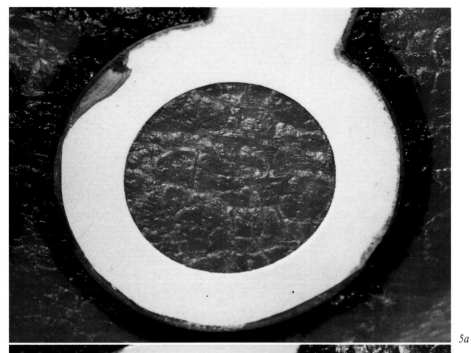

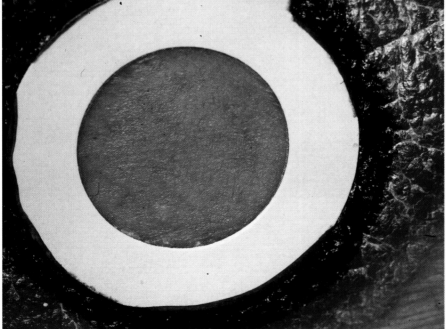
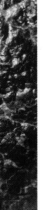

Psoriasis Plaque Test and Topical Corticosteroids

Plate III

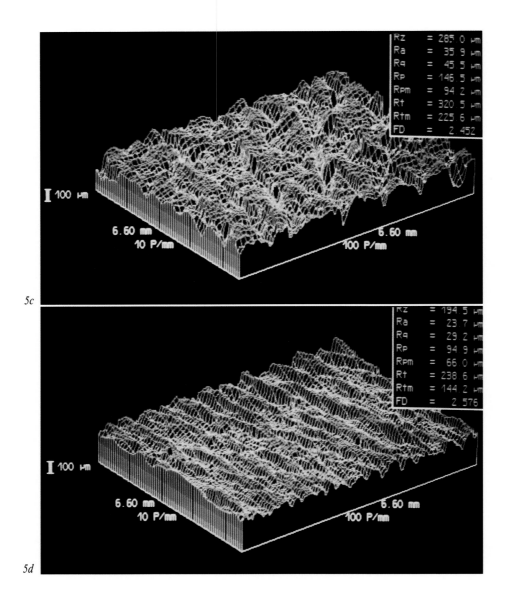

5c

5d

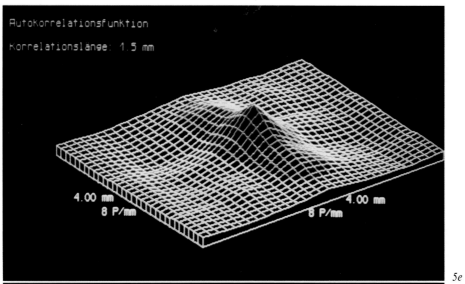

5e

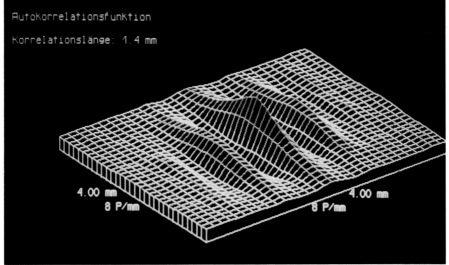

5f

(For legend see p. 112.)

of 'roughness' and 'irregularity', respectively 'smoothness' and 'regularity' of the skin. The method appears to be of value also for the analysis of other medical problems related to surface structures, for example of implants in dentistry and osteosynthetic materials in orthopedics.

In the case of the psoriasis plaque test, the results of the computerized laser profilometry show good correlation with the visual/sensory scores. It remains still open whether the quantitative data (roughness parameters) and the results of advanced mathematical evaluation (autocorrelation, power spectra) may improve the accuracy of the test by reliably discriminating even small differences in the therapeutic effects of different corticosteroids.

References

1   Wendt H, Frosch PJ: Clinicopharmacological Models for the Assay of Topical Corticoids. Basel, Karger, 1982.
2   Behrendt H, Korting HC: Klinische Prüfung von erwünschten und unerwünschten Wirkungen topisch applizierbarer Glukokortikosteroide am Menschen. Hautarzt 1990;41:2–8.
3   Dumas KJ, Scholz JR: The psoriasis bioassay for topical corticosteroid activity. Acta Derm Venerol (Stockh) 1972;52:43–48.
4   Schmeller W, Koch EMW, Wolff HH: Vergleichsprüfungen von Formulierungen mit steroidalen und nichtsteroidalen Wirkstoffen im Psoriasis-Plaque-Test. Z Hautkr 1986;61(suppl 2):87–96.
5   Wozel G, Barth J: Amcinonid und Prednicarbat. Vergleichende Untersuchung im Psoriasis-Plaque-Test. Akt Dermatol 1992;18:116–118.
6   Orfanos C: Die Oberfläche der Haut und ihrer Anhangsgebilde im Stereoelektronenmikroskop. Krankhafte Veränderungen und Einwirkungen exogener Noxen. Arch Derm Forsch 1972:244:80–85.
7   Nakayama Y, Kawasaki K, Kumagai H, Kaneko O, Mitsui T: Application of image analysis to the study of skin surface microtopography in relation to aging. J Appl Cosmetol 1986;4:97–110.
8   Marshall RJ, Marks R: Assessment of skin surface by scanning densitometry of macrophotographs. Clin Exp Dermatol 1987;8:121–127.
9   Gerrard WA: Friction and other measurements of the skin surface. Bioeng Skin 1987;3:123–139.
10   Makki S, Mignot J, Nadvornik IM, Agache P: Statistical analysis of human skin microtopographical profiles. Med Biol Eng Comput 1983;23:257–269.
11   Hoppe U, Lunderstädt R, Sauermann G: Quantitative Analyse der Hautoberfläche mit Hilfe der digitalen Signalverarbeitung. Ärztl Kosmetol 1986;16:13–37.
12   Nissen HP, Biltz H, Kreysel HW: Profilometrie, eine Methode zur Beurteilung der therapeutischen Wirksamkeit von Kamillosan-Salbe. Z Hautkr 1987;63:184–190.
13   Saur R, Schramm U, Steinhoff R, Wolff HH: Strukturanalyse der Hautoberfläche durch computergestützte Laser-Profilometrie. Hautarzt 1991;42:499–506.
14   Thomas RT (ed): Rough Surfaces. London, Longman, 1982.

Prof. Dr. H.H. Wolff, Dermatological Clinic, Medical University,
Ratzeburger Allee 160, D–23538 Lübeck (FRG)

Korting HC, Maibach HI (eds): Topical Glucocorticoids with Increased Benefit/Risk Ratio.
Curr Probl Dermatol. Basel, Karger, 1993, vol 21, pp 114–121

....

Topical Glucocorticoids and Thinning of Normal Skin as to Be Assessed by Ultrasound

Hans Christian Korting

Dermatologische Klinik und Poliklinik (Direktor: Prof. Dr. *G. Plewig*) der
Ludwig-Maximilians-Universität München, BRD

The introduction of topical hydrocortisone into the treatment of inflammatory skin disease has proven as a major breakthrough [1]. From the start on, however, it was clear that hydrocortisone could not be used successfully in the various existing types of inflammatory skin disease and that even in its prime indication, i.e. atopic eczema, efficacy was limited [1]. Before that background it again meant a breakthrough in dermatotherapy when Smith et al. [2] could report on the high efficacy of a fluorinated new compound of glucocorticoid character, i.e. triamcinolone acetonide. Yet it took only a few years to find out that increased efficacy of triamcinolone acetonide was also paralleled by severe adverse events: in 1963, Epstein et al. [3] described 'atrophic striae in patients with inguinal intertrigo'. Striae in fact can be considered as an overt and permanent type of skin atrophy which today is 'recognized as a most common adverse effect' [4]. The fear of both systemic and topic adverse events due to the application of topical glucocorticoids has during the last decades changed the focus of chemists insofar as no longer more potent but safer topical glucocorticoids are the key issue. The wish to obtain a glucocorticoid with an efficacy at least as high as the one of triamcinolone acetonide or rather the one of the later congener betamethasone-17-valerate [5] but with decreased unwanted effects, led to the development of the nonhalogenated but double-esterified compounds (i.e., prednicarbate or prednisolone-17-ethyl-carbonate-21-propionate) [6]. The general properties of this compound have been recently reviewed [7]. Later on, similar compounds have also been derived from hydrocortisone instead of prednisolone, e.g., hydrocortisone aceponate [8]. In this context it is of major interest to find out if such medium potent topical glucocorticoids indeed induce less skin thickness reduction as compared to classical compounds such as betamethasone-17-valerate or triamcinolone acetonide. As early as in 1981, ultrasound analysis has been proven successful to evaluate this particular facet of topical glucocorticoids [9]. With prednicarbate, however, so far conflicting evidence has been forwarded as to the potential for skin thickness reduction. While according to Dykes et al. [10] prednicarbate 0.25% cream applied openly does not reduce skin thickness more than the corresponding vehicle, this is claimed by Lubach and Grüter [11] who believe prednicarbate to be as potent in this respect as amcinonide. To answer the question definitely, the present investigation was performed. Moreover, hydrocortisone aceponate was tested in a trial of identical design to demonstrate that the reduction of atrophy potential of a medium potent glucocorticoid is not confined to just one particular compound, if present at all.

Materials and Methods

This is a report on two double-blind controlled trials of identical type except for some of the trial preparations. The design was approved by the local ethical committee and complied to the requirements of the Declaration of Helsinki. In each trial, 24 healthy adult volunteers applied two out of a total of four different glucocorticoid or base preparations.

In the first trial the four treatments were as follows: (A) 0.25% prednicarbate cream; (B) corresponding vehicle (cream base composed of paraffin oil, octyldodecanol, polysorbate 60, sorbitan monostearate, lactic acid, edetic acid, purified water, benzyl alcohol and stearic acid); (C) 0.1% betamethasone-17-valerate cream, and (D) 0.05% clobetasol-17-propionate cream.

In the second trial the four treatments were as follows: (A) hydrocortisone aceponate ointment 0.1%; (B) corresponding vehicle; (C) prednicarbate ointment 0.25%, and (D) betamethasone-17-valerate ointment 0.1%.

Either preparation A or B was to be applied to one forearm and preparation C or D to the other of each subject following a partially balanced incomplete block design. Allocation to the arms was at random. Accordingly, each treatment modality was applied to the right forearm of 6 and the left forearm of 6 additional volunteers. Twice daily, i.e., in the morning and in the evening, about 0.1 g of the test preparation was applied to the most proximal part of the flexor side of the forearm (close to the elbow), the area amounting to 4 × 4 cm. The test area was not covered for the first 10 min and not cleansed during the 2 h to follow. The entire treatment period comprised 6 weeks. Analysis of test sites consisted of visual inspection addressing signs of atrophy such as skin thinning, teleangiectasia and dryness (exsiccation). Moreover, ultrasound was used for assessing skin thickness. The points of time for analysis were the following: days 0 (before treatment), 4, 7, 14, 21, 28, 35, 42 (end of treatment) and 63 (follow-up). Treatment was to be discontinued immediately in case of clinical signs of atrophy or if skin thickness reduction as measured by ultrasound exceeded 40%.

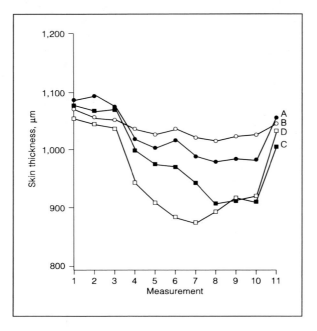

Fig. 1. Development of skin thickness upon twice daily open application of (A) predni-carbate 0.25% cream (●); (B) corresponding vehicle (○); (C) betamethasone-17-valerate 0.1% cream (■), and (D) clobetasol-17-propionate 0.1% cream (□), according to ultrasound analysis measurements 1, 2 and 3 being performed before application, 4–10 during application and 11 3 weeks afterwards. [From 12, with permission.]

For ultrasound analysis the DUB 20 system (Taberna pro medicum, Lüneburg, FRG) was used allowing both A- and B-scans. The system is composed of an applicator with a 20-MHz transducer (straight line 12.8 mm), a 20-MB personal computer for storage of 10 images each on a 1.2-MB floppy disk and a monitor with the resolution of 640 × 480 pixels providing pseudo-color images with 256 different shades. The straight line of 12.8 mm investigated was located in the center of the test area lying parallel to the axis of the forearm. Axial resolution amounted to 8 mm. First a representative B-mode image was viewed and thus five different spots selected to analyze skin thickness by itself using A-mode images. Skin thickness was defined as the thickness of both epidermis and corium together.

For statistical analysis first mean values and standard deviation were calculated. Thereafter the data of the first trial were subjected to bivariate analysis for independent samples. With the second trial, analysis of variance was performed. For parallelized comparisons of treatment modalities the error variance of the analysis of variance was used. Multiple testing of treatments followed the procedure of Bonferroni-Holm. In general, $p < 0.05$ was to be considered indicative of a difference. Additional information on the two trials can be obtained elsewhere [12, 13].

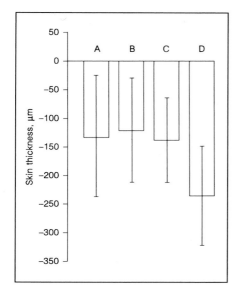

Fig. 2. Skin thickness reduction (mean value ± SD) upon 6 weeks' open application of (A) hydrocortisone aceponate 0.1% ointment; (B) corresponding vehicle; (C) prednicarbate 0.25% ointment, and (D) betamethasone-17-valerate 0.1% ointment. [From 13, with permission.]

Results

In general, there was no major difference in terms of skin thickness at the sites investigated before treatment. Skin thickness, however, changed a lot in the presence of some of the preparations investigated. Mean values for the various preparations within the first trial are given in figure 1. Hints at a difference in a statistical sense were seen with the following pairs of trial preparations as early as on day 21: A vs. D, B vs. C, B vs. D, and C vs. D.

Corresponding results were found in the second trial. Figure 2 gives the mean values as well as standard deviations for skin thickness after 6 weeks' application of the various trial preparations. Figures 3 and 4 demonstrate a B-mode image before the application of betamethasone-17-valerate and after 6 weeks' application. A corresponding set of images for prednicarbate is represented by figures 5 and 6.

In the first trial the application of one trial preparation, i.e., clobetasol-17-propionate, had to be stopped before the time scheduled. In 1 individual this was the case on day 14 and in 9 on day 21. In all cases except 1 this was due to severe dryness (exsiccation), once initial teleangiectasia and striae distensae were observed which, however, proved reversible thereafter.

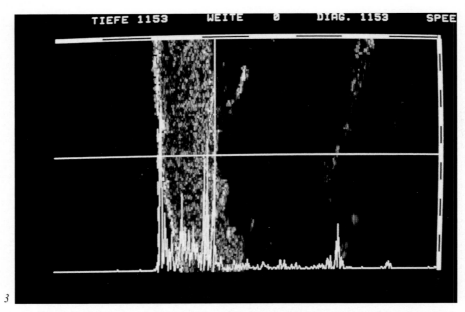

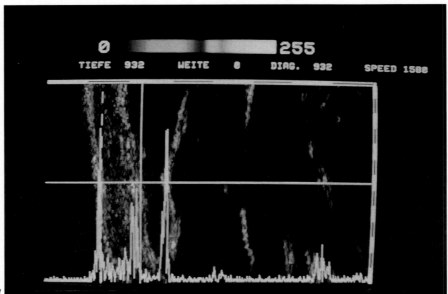

Fig. 3. B-mode image of human skin before daily application of betamethasone-17-valerate ointment for 6 weeks.

Fig. 4. B-mode image of human skin after twice daily application of betamethasone-17-valerate ointment for 6 weeks.

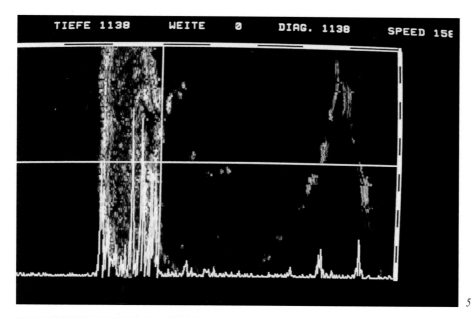

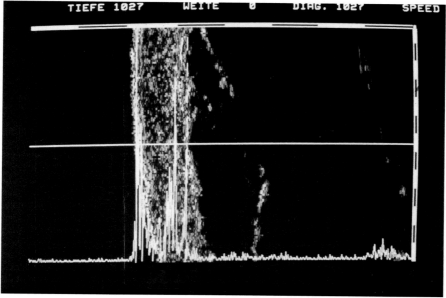

Fig. 5. B-mode image of human skin before application of prednicarbate ointment for 6 weeks.

Fig. 6. B-mode image of human skin after twice daily application of prednicarbate ointment for 6 weeks.

Discussion

According to the present results there is a marked difference in terms of the skin thinning potential of convential medium potent and highly potent halogenated glucocorticoids as represented by betamethasone-17-valerate and clobetasol-17-propionate. With nonhalogenated glucocorticoids of the double-ester type as represented by prednicarbate and hydrocortisone aceponate, a skin thickness reduction is also seen which, however, only lies in the order of magnitude also observed with corresponding vehicles. Thus there is a clear difference in the pertinent activity of topical glucocorticoid compounds. Findings concerning both prednicarbate and betamethasone-17-valerate do not differ according to the vehicle, i.e. if either cream or ointment is used.

The data suggest that there is a clear difference in terms of the benefit-risk ratio of medium potent topical glucocorticoids given that betamethasone-17-valerate and both prednicarbate and hydrocortisone aceponate are actually alike in terms of the anti-inflammatory potential. The findings concerning prednicarbate in particular confirm previous findings by Dykes et al. [10] using the A-mode only. They are in clear contrast to the findings by Lubach and Grüter [11].

Ultrasound analysis using both the B- and A-mode has proven helpful in the characterization of the safety profile of various topical glucocorticoids.

Data as obtained here in connection with data on the anti-inflammatory activity as to be obtained using human assays such as the UV-erythema test should enable us to question conventional wisdom according to which 'different topical glucocorticosteroids ... differ only in potency' [14]. In the longer term the increase of the benefit-risk ratio of topical glucocorticoids could have a major impact on treatment protocols in clinical practice.

Acknowledgments

I am grateful to Dr. Th. Höhler and K. Wörz, Cassella-Riedel Pharma GmbH, Frankfurt, FRG, as well as Dr. F. Rippke, Beiersdorf AG, Hamburg, FRG, and Dr. K. Schnitker from Bielefeld, FRG, for providing the test preparations and for statistical analysis.

References

1   Sulzberger MB, Witten VH: Effect of topically applied compound F in selected dermatoses. J Invest Dermatol 1952;19:101–102.
2   Smith JG Jr, Zawisza J, Blank H: Triamcinolone acetonide: Highly effective new topical steroid. Arch Dermatol 1958;78:643–645.
3   Epstein NN, Epstein WL, Epstein JH: Atrophic striae in patients with inguinal intertrigo. Arch Dermatol 1963;87:450–457.

4   Kligman AM: Adverse effects of topical corticosteroids; in Christophers E, Schöpf E, Kligman AM, Stoughton RB (eds): Topical Corticosteroid Therapy. A Novel Approach to Safer Drugs. New York, Raven Press, 1988, pp 181–187.

5   Samson C, Peets E, Winter-Sperry R, Wolkoff A: Betamethasone-valerate – Valisone® – establishment of a new standard for topical corticosteroid potency; in Maibach HI, Surber C (eds): Topical Corticosteroids. Basel, Karger, 1992, pp 335–348.

6   Stache U, Alpermann HG: Zur Chemie und Pharmakologie von Prednicarbat (Hoe 777), einem halogenfreien, topisch anti-inflammatorisch wirksamen Derivat des Prednisolon-17-ethylkohlensäureesters. Z Hautkr 1986;61 (suppl 1):3–6.

7   Drebinger K, Hoehler T: Prednicarbate; in Maibach HI, Surber C (eds): Topical Corticosteroids. Basel, Karger, 1992, pp 480–493.

8   Flasch CI, Klaschka F: Therapeutisches Profil des ersten Hydrocortisondiesters in lipophiler Grundlage. Dtsch Dermatol 1986;7:806–828.

9   Tan C, Marks R, Payne P: Comparison of xeroradiographic and ultrasound detection of corticosteroid induced dermal thinning. J Invest Dermatol 1981;76:126–128.

10 Dykes PJ, Hill S, Marks R: Assessment of the atrophogenicity potential of corticosteroids by ultrasound by epidermal biopsy under occlusive and non-occlusive conditions; in Christophers E, Schöpf E, Kligman AM, Stoughton RB (eds): Topical Corticosteroid Therapy. A Novel Approach to Safer Drugs. New York, Raven Press, 1988, pp 111–118.

11 Lubach D, Grüter M: Vergleichende Untersuchungen über die hautverdünnende Wirkung von Amcinonid und Prednicarbat an unterschiedlichen Körperregionen des Menschen. Akt Dermatol 1988;14:197–200.

12 Korting HC, Vieluf D, Kerscher M: 0.25% prednicarbate cream and the corresponding vehicle induce less skin atrophy than 0.1% betamethasone-17-valerate cream and 0.05% clobetasol-17-propionate cream. Eur J Clin Pharmacol 1992;42:159–161.

13 Kerscher MJ, Korting HC: Topical glucocorticoids of the non-fluorinated double-ester type. Lack of atrophogenicity in normal skin as assessed by high-frequency ultrasound. Acta Derm Venereol (Stockh) 1992;72:214–216.

14 Shuster S: Eczema; in Greaves MW, Shuster S (eds): Pharmacology of the Skin. Berlin, Springer, 1989, vol II, pp 439–445.

Prof. Hans C. Korting, MD, Dermatologische Klinik und Poliklinik der Ludwig-Maximilians-Universität, Frauenlobstrasse 9-11, D–80337 München (FRG)

Korting HC, Maibach HI (eds): Topical Glucocorticoids with Increased Benefit/Risk Ratio.
Curr Probl Dermatol. Basel, Karger, 1993, vol 21, pp 122–131

....

Side Effects of Topical Glucocorticoids

C.M. Mills, R. Marks

Department of Dermatology, University Hospital of Wales, Cardiff, UK

Topical steroids have a complex anti-inflammatory action, although the entire mechanisms by which they exert this effect are not fully understood. Glucocorticoid molecules bind to the steroid receptor molecules on the cell membrane and then the steroid-receptor complex diffuses into the nucleus and alters gene expression and mRNA synthesis which in turn modifies cell activity [1]. A particularly important aspect of glucocorticoid activity is the induction of changes in production of endogenous inhibitors of lipo-oxygenases, i.e. the lipocortins [2], leading in turn to decreased production of inflammatory eicosanoids. The synthesis of several cytokines is reduced, including interleukin-1, which in turn alters inflammatory cell chemotaxis and increases vascular tone causing vasoconstriction. This latter effect is exploited in the vasoconstrictor test of steroid potency. Glucocorticoids also reduce the mitotic rate of keratinocytes [3] and, therefore, the population of cells in the epidermis causing decreased epidermal thickness. They also bring about a reduction in epidermal cell size which contributes to the reduction in thickness of the epidermis. This action is partially responsible for the effects of skin thinning; however, the main effect causing this side effect is on the dermis. Topical steroids reduce the numbers of fibroblasts in the dermis as well as impairing their function by diminishing the production of collagen and proteoglycans [4].

Clinical Features

Systemic Effects

Pituitary adrenal axis suppression is a potentially life-threatening side effect which may occur with the use of topical as well as systemically administered steroids. The degree of adrenal suppression is dependent on many factors including the duration of treatment, the strength of steroid used, the area of skin to which the steroid is applied as well as the condition of the skin. The amount of topical steroid required to produce adrenal suppression will vary between patients but may be as little as 50 g/week of a steroid such as 0.05% clobetasol propionate. Excessive use of potent topical steroids may also result in iatrogenic Cushing's disease. Patients may develop a low serum potassium level, diabetes mellitus, hypertension and osteoporosis. Systemic effects are particularly important in paediatric practice where growth development may be suppressed by overzealous use of potent topical steroids.

Local Side Effects

Dermal Thinning. Cutaneous thinning (skin atrophy) is perhaps the best known adverse event following treatment with topical steroids. Atrophic skin appears smooth, shiny and pink (fig. 1). The vessels becoming more prominent as the overlying skin thins. The thinning is due to reduction in the rate of synthesis of the protein constituents of the dermis. This can be quantified in a number of ways, to assess the atrophogenic potential of new topical steroids.

Reduction of collagen and supporting tissue leads to striae distensae which are a cosmetically undesirable side effect. Striae tend to occur around the flexures, and are initially bright pink or lurid pink/purplish in colour. This process is not reversible although the striae do shrink and fade to become thinner and paler with time (striae albicantes) with some degree of cosmetic improvement.

Bruising following minimal trauma or spontaneously is a feature frequently seen with the use of topical steroids and is also attributable to loss of perivascular supporting tissue. The resulting intradermal haemorrhage spreads easily. Marked telangectasia are associated with prolonged use of steroids producing a ruddy appearance particularly when on the face. Corticosteroids may also produce vasoconstriction and pale skin, although how this occurs is uncertain.

Masked Infection. Topical steroids may mask and alter the expression of several common skin disorders. Dermatophyte infection of the skin causes an eczematous reaction in which the infected superficial layers of the skin become inflamed and are shed, so clearing the organism. However, if topical steroids are used on these patients, the anti-inflammatory effects of steroids will suppress this response leading to a more protracted and more extensive condition. This is known as tinea incognito. Bacterial infections such as impetigo, a superficial skin infection due to either staphylococci or streptococci, may also be potentiated by treatment with topical steroids as may viral infections such as eczema herpeticum.

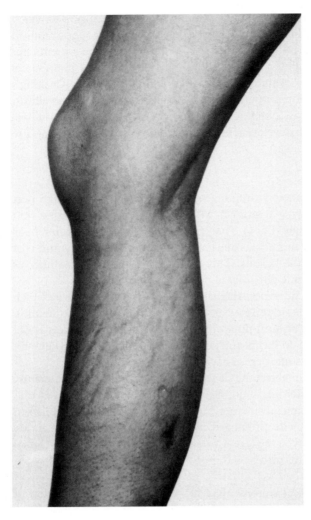

Fig. 1. Lower leg of woman who had used potent topical corticosteroids for some time on this area showing the development of striae. Note also the vascular markings which are easily seen because of the skin thinning.

Conditions Associated with Topical Steroid Usage. Some conditions are recognized as the direct sequelae of the use of topical steroids. Perioral dermatitis is a micropapulo-pustular eruption often thought to be induced by the use of topical steroids on the skin around the mouth and chin. This condition usually occurs in females and responds to oral tetracyclines and withdrawal of the corticosteroid.

Steroids are sometimes inappropriately used in conditions such as acne and rosacea, which may flare dramatically after steroid withdrawal. Rosacea is in particular aggravated by the use of corticosteroid topically and patients may develop a beacon-like red face. Hirsuties and localized areas of hypertrichosis are also recognized complications of topical steroids, although uncommon and rarely troublesome.

Withdrawal of Steroids. Sudden cessation of treatment with topical steroids may also cause adverse events such as the rebound phenomena seen in psoriasis when withdrawal of steroids may exacerbate psoriasis, and even result in a generalized pustular form of the disease.

Allergy. Allergic contact dermatitis has been reported with the use of some topical steroids although this is uncommon. It is always important to distinguish between a reaction to the glucocorticoid or to a component of the vehicle cream. Care must be taken in the selection of preparations used in patients with known hypersensitivities. Propylene glycol, cetostearyl alcohol and parabens (hydroxybenzoates) are the most frequent sensitizers encountered. Glucocorticoid preparations may also contain antibiotics such as neomycin, which also frequently causes skin sensitization.

Measurement of Side Effects

Methods for assessing the damage induced by treatments such as corticosteroids are essential and should ideally be predictive, simple and reproducible. Much work has been performed in the past using animal studies. We believe that these tests have limited value due to differences in the structure of animal skin compared with human skin as well as differing metabolism and actions of topical steroids in animals compared with humans. Many in vitro tests have also been proposed but the pharmacokinetics and the in vivo tissue interactions are so important that these also have limited predictive value in our view.

One simple human in vivo method for assessing skin thinning is by measuring the thickness of whole skin with skin calipers (e.g. Harpenden skin fold calipers) [5]. This is the most direct, simple method of determining the skin thickness but although a useful guide, individual readings have a low degree of reliability. The calipers measure predominantly dermal thickness but include the epidermis and may also pick up fat. In addition, compressive forces are difficult to avoid using this method. X-ray measurements of the skin provide more accurate quantification of skin thickness, but the disadvantage of this method is that of exposing the patient to ionizing radiation [6]. A safer method of estimating thinning of the skin is by using ultrasound. Ultrasound measurement of the skin using a pulsed A-scan device with transducers in the 15–20 MHz range are particularly useful for this purpose. The ultrasound device measures the time difference between the signal returning from the skin surface and the dermal fat. As the speed of sound through skin is known then the distance (thickness) of the skin can be calculated. This method is safe, simple, accurate and reproducible.

Study Design

We have used ultrasound and superficial skin surface biopsies in many studies to determine the degree of skin atrophy following application of both widely used topical steroid preparations and novel formulations in development including prednicarbate. This is a novel corticosteroid designed to possess potent anti-inflammatory properties without cutaneous atrophy. Normal volunteer subjects with no history of skin disease or recent corticosteroid therapy were recruited for these studies. Informed witnessed consent was obtained from all volunteer subjects. Ethical approval for the study was obtained from the University Hospital of Wales/College of Medicine.

Skin thickness was measured by pulsed A-scan ultrasound using a Dermal Depth Detector (Dermtronics Ltd, Cardiff, UK) [7]. Results are expressed in microseconds, and the conversion factor 1 μs = 0.79 mm. No attempt was made to distinguish between epidermis and dermis and the measurement is of epidermal plus dermal thickness = skin thickness. A minimum of 5 measurements were taken at each site.

Superficial skin surface biopsies were taken by stripping with cyanoacrylate adhesives. These were fixed in formalin and processed by routine histological methods. Sections were prepared, stained with haematoxylin and eosin, and the mean epidermal thickness (MET) and mean keratinocyte height (MKH) determined using an Optimax V image analysis system (Synoptics, UK) [8].

Study 1 – Cutaneous Atrophy under Occlusion

A total of 12 male subjects (age range 24–55 years, mean age 36 years) took part in this study. Each of the subjects was treated with the following six materials: (1) 0.25% prednicarbate cream; (2) cream vehicle (placebo control); (3) 1% hydrocortisone cream; (4) 0.1% hydrocortisone-17-butyrate cream; (5) 0.1% betamethasone-17-valerate cream, and (6) 0.05% clobetasol propionate cream.

Approximately 0.1 g of each of the materials was applied to the forearm using 12 mm aluminium Finn chambers on Scanpor tape. The test materials were allocated in a random fashion to 6 treatment sites on the forearm (6 sites/arm). The materials were renewed 3 times weekly for a period of 4 weeks. Assessment of skin

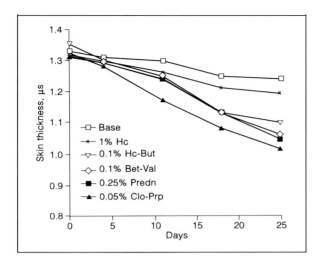

Fig. 2. Study 1 – occlusive application: The change in skin thickness as measured by ultrasound versus duration of study. Results expressed as μs (1 μs = 0.79 mm). 1% Hc = 1% hydrocortisone; 0.1% Hc-But = 0.1% hydrocortisone-17-butyrate; 0.1% Bet-Val = 0.1% betamethasone-17-valerate; 0.25% Predn = 0.25% prednicarbate; 0.05% Clo-Prp = 0.05% clobetasol propionate.

thickness was made using pulsed A-scan ultrasound at days 0, 4, 11, 18 and 25 of the study.

Statistical Analysis. In order to avoid any assumptions about the normality of the data derived from these experiments, nonparametric methods of analysis were used. The Friedman two-way analysis of variance was used in the situation where each subject received all possible treatments. Where subjects only received some of the treatments, the Durbin test for balanced incomplete blocks design was used. This test was reduced to a Friedman test when the number of treatments equals the number of experimental units per block. The Friedman and Durbin tests are described in Conover [9].

Results. As would be expected, potent corticosteroids such as 0.1% betamethasone-17-valerate and 0.05% clobetasol propionate produced marked atrophy of the skin with a reduction of approximately 20% over the 25-day period (fig. 2). On the other hand, 1% hydrocortisone, a weak corticosteroid, gave a reduction of approximately 3%, which was not different from base alone. The 0.1% hydrocortisone-17-butyrate produced a moderate degree of atrophy, intermediate between hydrocortisone and the more potent corticosteroids. A new corticosteroid, 0.25%

Table 1. Study 2 – occlusive application of corticosteroids

Treatment	Mean epidermal thickness µm ± SD, n = 10	Mean keratinocyte height µm ± SD, n = 10
Base	53.40 ± 9.06	9.97 ± 1.07
1% hydrocortisone	46.84 ± 11.34	10.13 ± 1.17
0.1% hydrocortisone-17-butyrate	28.83 ± 4.06	9.23 ± 1.14
0.1% betamethasone-17-valerate	29.46 ± 5.56	9.24 ± 1.26
0.25% predicarbate	27.83 ± 4.03	9.15 ± 0.88
0.05% clobetasol propionate	29.76 ± 6.95	9.57 ± 1.31

prednicarbate, produced levels of atrophy comparable to the most potent corticosteroids. A statistical analysis of the values at day 25 indicated the following statistically significant differences at $p < 0.05$: (a) base was significantly different from 0.25% prednicarbate, 0.1% hydrocortisone-17-butyrate, 0.1% betamethasone-17-valerate, and 0.05% clobetasol propionate; (b) the 1% hydrocortisone was significantly different from 0.25% prednicarbate, 0.1% betamethasone-17-valerate, and 0.05% clobetasol propionate; (c) the 0.1% hydrocortisone-17-butyrate was significantly different from 0.05% clobetasol propionate.

Study 2 – Epidermal Atrophy under Occlusion

A total of 30 subjects, 11 male and 19 female (age range 19–55 years, mean age 34 years), took part in this study. Each of the subjects was treated with 2 out of the 6 materials as listed above. The test materials were applied to the forearms, 1 per forearm, under occlusion as above. Allocation of treatments was by a balanced, incomplete blocks design such that each treatment appeared 10 times. The test materials were renewed 3 times weekly for a period of 4 weeks. At the end of this period, superficial skin biopsies were taken and processed as above for estimation of MET and MKH.

Results. The results of study 2 are presented in table 1. The results for MET in general parallel the results for skin thickness measurements. As found in study 1, 0.25% prednicarbate produced the same degree of epidermal atrophy as the more potent corticosteroids such as 0.1% betamethasone-17-valerate. The results for MKH did not show significant differences between treatments.

A statistical analysis of the MET data indicated the following statistically significant differences at $p < 0.05$: (a) base was significantly different from 0.25% prednicarbate, 0.1% hydrocortisone-17-butyrate, 0.1% betamethasone-17-valerate, and 0.05% clobetasol propionate; (b) the 1% hydrocortisone was significantly different from 0.025% prednicarbate.

A statistical analysis of the MKH data indicated no significant differences between treatments at p = 0.05.

Study 3 – Cutaneous and Epidermal Atrophy with No Occlusion
A total of 25 subjects, 5 male and 19 female (age range 19–54 years, mean age 33 years), took part in this study. Each of the subjects was treated with 2 out of the following 4 materials: (1) 0.25% prednicarbate cream; (2) 0.025% fluocinolone acetonide; (3) 0.1% betamethasone-17-valerate, and (4) prednicarbate base.

Treatments were randomly allocated using a balanced, incomplete blocks design such that treatment was replicated 12 times. Materials were applied to an area of 8 × 5 cm at a dose of 10 mg/cm^2 without occlusion. Applications were made twice daily over an 8-week period. Skin thickness measurements were made at 0, 7, 14, 21, 28, 35, 42, 49 and 56 days. At the end of the study period, superficial skin biopsies were taken and processed for estimation of MET and MKH, as above.

Results. The results of the nonocclusive study are presented in fig. 3 and table 2. The application of 0.1% betamethasone-17-valerate and 0.025% fluocinolone acetonide produced marked atrophy in this study. In contrast, 0.25% prednicarbate did not differ from the base vehicle in terms of its effect on skin thickness. A statistical analysis on the data at day 56 indicated that the following differences were significant at p < 0.05: (a) base was significantly different from 0.1% betamethasone-17-valerate and 0.025% fluocinolone acetonide; (b) the 0.25% prednicarbate was significantly different from 0.1% betamethasone-17-valerate and 0.025% flucinolone acetonide.

The results of the MET measurements (table 2) parallel the ultrasound readings. A statistical analysis of the data indicated that the following differences were significant at p < 0.05: (a) base was significantly different from 0.1% betamethasone-17-valerate and 0.025% fluocinolone acetonide; (b) the 0.25% prednicarbate was significantly different from 0.025% fluocinolone acetonide.

The results for MKH readings did not show significant differences between treatments. A statistical analysis indicated no statistically significant differences at p = 0.05.

Conclusions

Prednicarbate is a novel corticosteroid designed to possess potent anti-inflammatory properties without the commonly occurring side effects such as cutaneous atrophy. Early studies in the rat [10] indicated that prednicarbate

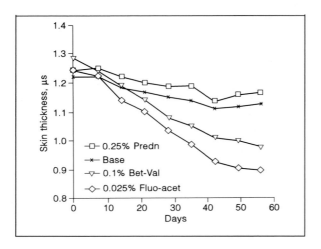

Fig. 3. Study 3 – nonocclusive application: The change in skin thickness as measured by ultrasound versus duration of study. Results expressed as µs (1 µs = 0.79 mm). 0.25% Predn = 0.25% prednicarbate; 0.1% Bet-Val = 0.1% betamethasone-17-valerate; 0.025% Fluo-acet = 0.025% fluocinolone acetonide.

Table 2. Study 3 – nonocclusive application of corticosteroids

Treatment	Mean epidermal thickness µm ± SD	Mean keratinocyte height µm ± SD
Base	49.42±5.21	11.64±0.93
0.25% prednicarbate	46.73±4.66	11.39±0.84
0.1% betamethasone-17-valerate	41.52±4.50	11.31±0.81
0.025% fluocinolone acetonide	38.40±7.80	11.69±0.63

applied topically without occlusion did not inhibit collagen synthesis or produce dermal atrophy. The studies reported here show that in normal volunteer human subjects, nonocclusive application of 0.25% prednicarbate has a similar lack of effect on cutaneous atrophy. This contrasts with the occlusive study also reported here, where 0.25% prednicarbate produced a similar degree of atrophy as 0.1% betamethasone-17-valerate and 0.05% clobetasol propionate. The reasons for difference in side effects in the occlusive and nonocclusive situations are not completely clear. The most likely explanation is a variation in the rate of penetration of prednicarbate and its subsequent rate of biotransformation. However, the lack of atrophogenicity in clinical studies, where the stratum corneum barrier function is compromised, indicates that other factors may well be involved.

The results of the measurements of epidermal atrophy in the nonocclusive and occlusive studies indicate that the sparing effect of prednicarbate is not restricted to the dermis. Thus, the epidermal atrophy induced by 0.25% prednicarbate in the nonocclusive study was not significantly different from base control.

The studies reported here show that 0.25% prednicarbate does not produce significant dermal or epidermal atrophy when applied nonocclusively in normal human subjects over an 8-week period.

Topical steroids are an essential part of the dermatologist's armoury for dealing with skin disease. The side effects are well known and well recognized, with new products continually being sought that will combine the efficacy of a potent topical steroid and yet not lead to harmful side effects with prolonged use. It is essential that accurate means of measuring the potency and atrophogenicity of topical glucocorticosteroids are available in dermatology and we would recommend the use of pulsed A-scan ultrasound for this purpose.

References

1 Yohn JJ, Weston WL: Topical glucocorticoids; in Weston (ed): Current Problems in Dermatology, vol 11/2. Chicago, Year Book Medical Publishers, 1990.
2 Di Rosa M, Flowers RJ, Hiratu F, et al: Antiphospholipid proteins. Prostaglandins 1984;28:441–442.
3 Fischer LB, Maubach HI: The effect of corticosteroids on human epidermal mitotic activity. Arch Dermatol 1971;103:39.
4 Saarni H, Tammi M, Doherty NS: Decreased hyaluronic acid synthesis, a sensitive indicator of cortisol action. J Pharmacol 1978;30:200–201.
5 Booth RAD, Goddard BA, Paton A: Measurement of fat thickness in man: A comparison of ultrasound, Harpenden calipers and electrical conductivity. Br J Nutr 1966;20:719–725.
6 Tan CY, Statham B, Marks R, Payne PA: Comparison of xeroradiographic and ultrasound detection of corticosteroid-induced damage. J Invest Dermatol 1982;716:126–128.
7 Pearce AD, Gaskell SH, Marks R: Epidermal changes in human skin following irradiation with either UVA or UVB. J Invest Dermatol 1987;88:83–87.
8 Tan CY, Statham B, Marks R, Payne PA: Skin thickness measurement by pulsed ultrasound: Its reproducibility, validation and variability. Br J Dermatol 1982;106:657–667.
9 Conover WJ: Practical Nonparametric Statistics. ed 2. New York, Wiley, 1980.
10 Dipetrello T, Lee H, Cutroneo KH: Anti-inflammatory adrenal steroids that neither inhibit skin collagen synthesis or cause dermal atrophy. Arch Dermatol 1984;120:878–883.

Prof. R. Marks, Department of Dermatology, University Hospital of Wales, Heath Park, Cardiff CF4 4XW (UK)

Korting HC, Maibach HI (eds): Topical Glucocorticoids with Increased Benefit/Risk Ratio.
Curr Probl Dermatol. Basel, Karger, 1993, vol 21, pp 132–139

....

Early Detection of Glucocorticoid-Specific Epidermal Alterations Using Skin Surface Microscopy

H. Schulz[a], *K. H. Nietsch*[b], *Th. Höhler*[b]

[a] Dermatologische Praxis, Bergkamen;
[b] Cassella-Riedel Pharma GmbH, Frankfurt/Main, BRD

The topical application of glucocorticosteroids remains indispensable for the treatment of acute-stage noninfectious inflammatory dermatoses and of those with a tendency to chronicity or recurrence. In spite of intensive endeavors on the part of dermatologists to keep patients informed, skin-care-oriented treatment designs and the development of corticoids with an improved risk/benefit ratio [1–3], patients' fears regarding cortisone are, if anything, tending to increase. Ambivalence towards corticosteroid therapy is even widespread among prescribing physicians. Irrational fears can only be reduced by making knowledge more readily available and by reconciling physicians with the drug. Numerous test methods have been developed for evaluating local adverse effects of corticosteroids, e.g. the Duhring chamber test, ammonium hydroxide blister test, corticosteroid stratum corneum test, skin fold compression and thickness measurements, determination of transepidermal water loss, and skin thickness measurements by ultrasound. All these methods are costly in that they are time-consuming and requiring expensive equipment; they are used primarily for classifying corticosteroids of differing potencies. In some cases the tests are conducted under occlusive conditions, when a 10- to 100-fold increase in the biological activity of the substance can be anticipated [4].

Since 1988 attempts have been made to establish relevant criteria for evaluating adverse epidermal effects of corticosteroids under noninvasive and nonocclusive clinical conditions by using skin surface microscopy. A portable light microscope with a scale incorporated into the stage (a.d.n.-Medizintechnik, Hamm, FRG) was suitable for routine diagnosis. High-resolution skin surface photography as described by Bahmer and Rohrer [5] was used to document the findings.

In order to identify corticosteroid-induced atrophogenic skin changes, earlier hemilateral studies in which the substance was applied for periods of 6 months were now supplemented with a double-blind study in which two commercially available topical corticosteroids were tested. It seems that in the highly typical characteristics of an altered skin surface derived from the results of this study by structural analysis the treating physician will have at his or her disposal evaluation criteria for an accurate assessment of the severity of adverse effects and the risk of continuing the treatment, or for identifying any damage present, even before the application of the substance.

Subjects and Method

In a randomized, intraindividual, hemilateral double-blind comparative study lasting 6 months, two glucocorticoids of the same potency class III were investigated by topical application in 10 healthy volunteers. A healthy 39-year-old women (skin type II) left untreated with glucocorticoids served as control.

This trial was based on a design approved by the local ethical committee and complied with the requirements of the Helsinki declaration.

Five of the subjects were female and 5 were male. The median age was 28 (18–45) years. Two volunteers were of skin type I (low pigmentation), 4 were of skin type II, 3 had moderately pigmented skin (type III) and 1 had highly pigmented skin (type IV). The test substances were prednicarbate 0.25% (PC) and betamethasone 17-valerate 0.1% (BMV), two topical glucocorticoids of potency grade III [6], in an oil-in-water emulsion base. The control volunteer received the corresponding cream bases.

The application field was a 10×10 cm area of skin below the distal fold of the elbow. According to Feldmann and Maibach [7], the ventral skin of the forearm shows a relatively low penetration score (factor 1) for topical corticosteroids (cf. back 1.7, forehead 6.0). The advantages of using the volar forearm are good accessibility, slight covering of hair in most cases, easy application of the test substance and ideal comparability in the hemilateral test. This area is also the test region preferred by other investigators.

A strip of ointment 2 cm in length was applied once a day to the skin of both forearms and rubbed in. Compliance of the volunteer was monitored by regular weighings of the tube contents. The course of the clinical epidermal skin changes and those visible under a direct microscope was documented every 14 days to day 180. The clinical symptoms comprised the criteria redness, desquamation, burning and tenderness, using the scores 0 = absent, 1 = slight, 2 = moderate and 3 = severe. The symptoms regarded as characteristic of epidermal and dermal skin changes were distortion of the skin topography to form parallel striae, desquamation of the stratum corneum, telangiectasia, petechiae, loss of skin topography and ostiofollicular inflammation. This hierarchy was assigned scores of 1–6, with reference to the atrophogenic potency of the substance.

The skin signs were photographed by the method of Bahmer and Rohrer [5], using an Olympus camera system comprising an OM2 single-lens reflex camera, bellows, a 38-mm macro lens and a specially prepared stage with a bracket to take the flash unit. The primary magnification was $\times$ 5.5. For photographing, the upper edge of the stage was positioned medially in the distal fold in the bend of the elbow. Before application of the ointment began, the untreated skin fields on both forearms were photographed, before and after immersing in oil. The findings were evaluated statistically using descriptive p values, the Wilcoxon-Pratt test and a last value analysis. $p < 0.05$ was considered significant.

Results

The normal, finely furrowed skin surface consisted of raised, cushion-like fields which were rhombic, trapezoid or triangular in shape (fig. 1). The highest points within these fields showed delicate punctiform or thread-like capillaries which were particularly noticeable after immersing in oil. The first changes observed under the direct light microscope following local application of the test substances were distortion of the skin topography to form parallel striae, associated with a clearly recognizable loss of turgor of the normally plump, cushioned surface.

Since slight distortion of the skin into parallel striae was even observed in the control volunteer following long-term application of the cream bases, the dermal ridges caused by the distortion were measured. It was found that if the ridges were 130–200 µm apart the finding could be regarded as corticosteroid-independent, i.e. as corresponding to normal transepidermal water and turgor loss due to application of the cream base. In agreement with the results of earlier investigations [8], ridges less than 130 µm apart were attributable to glucocorticoid-specific atrophogenic effects. The measurements were made using a cross-wire graticule with rings at 0.4-mm intervals. If there were 4 or more ridges between the limits the effect was deemed to be glucocorticoid-specific. The phenomenon of distortion was less pronounced following immersion in oil. Only marked distortion into parallel striae was used for definitive statistical evaluation of the course control data during application of the active substance.

The slight changes appeared, on average, after 2 weeks (median 16.3 days) on the BMV side and after 4 weeks (median 28.6 days) on the PC side. Marked glucocorticoid-specific distortion into parallel striae occurred on average after 67 days of application of BMV, whereas under PC this phenomenon occurred within the 180-day period in only 2 of the 10 subjects, appearing in one of these volunteers (No. 2, male, skin type I) after 54 days and in the other (No. 6, female, skin type II) after 124 days.

Fig. 1. Normal skin surface of the flexor side of the forearm close to the elbow. $\times$ 5.5.
Fig. 2. Volunteer No. 6 after 180 days of BMV treatment. Pronounced parallel striae of the skin surface, partial destruction and telangiectasis are seen.

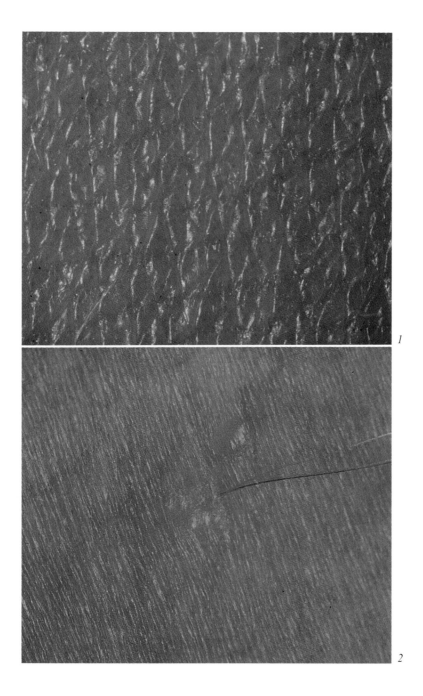

As an additional epidermal sign, desquamation of the corneum stratum due to loss of the horny layer was observed after BMV had been applied for on average 53 days. Only 3 volunteers showed desquamation on the side treated with PC, after 91 days on average (40–180 days). 2 of these were of skin type I and 1 was of skin type II.

The median time of onset of slight to fairly pronounced telangiectases on the BMV side was 108 days (82–153 days). On the PC side, slight telangiectases were observed in 1 volunteer of skin type I (No. 2) after 54 days. On the BMV side this man showed an increase in telangiectases after only 26 days.

Faint petechiae were observed in 1 subject (No. 10, male, skin type III); this symptom appeared on the BMV side after 171 days. Partial destruction of the skin topography was seen in 1 volunteer (No. 6, female, skin type II) after 180 days of use of BMV (fig. 2). In 1 subject (No. 8, female, skin type I), pronounced ostiofollicular inflammation was observed on the BMV side after 111 days. Isolated slightly inflamed follicles were seen on the BMV side in 2 subjects (No. 7, 10) after 124 days; yet a link with application of the substance appeared questionable.

The study was discontinued hemilaterally in 3 volunteers. No. 1, female, skin type II, discontinued use of the substance on the left forearm (BMV) after 148 days on account of severe skin redness, desquamation and tenderness. The microscopic findings were marked distortion with parallel striae, desquamation of the stratum corneum and telangiectases. No. 8 discontinued application of the substance on the right forearm (BMV) after 111 days on account of ostiofollicular inflammation and skin redness, and No. 10 terminated treatment of the right arm (BMV) after 171 days on account of severe erythema, desquamation and pruritus. The differences of the adverse effects between the BMV side and the PC side became significant from day 82 onward ($p < 0.05$; fig. 3). Regression of these unwanted symptoms began within 14 days in volunteer No. 10 and within 31 days in No. 1, but not until 69 days after discontinuation in No. 8.

Discussion

Numerous human pharmacological test models have been developed to evaluate the correlation between the main effects and side effects of topically applied glucocorticosteroids [9–14]. However, with all these methods, methodological and technical drawbacks of varying importance must be taken into account. In particular, the tests in the framework of dermatological clinical practice are of only limited usefulness and leave unanswered many questions of interest to the clinician. As regards treatment, it is of primary importance to know whether corticosteroids may be used under clinical conditions without a risk of permanent adverse skin changes and for how long in a given case.

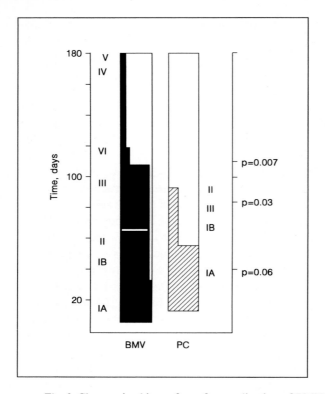

Fig. 3. Changes in skin surface after application of BMV and PC creams. IA = Slight parallel striae; IB = marked parallel striae; II = desquamation; III = telangiectases; IV = petechiae; V = partial destruction; VI = ostiofollicular inflammation.

Noninvasive mechanical methods for measuring skin folds [15] or for measuring compression or thickness [16, 17] are often difficult to use for quantitative analyses [18, 19]. From a frequency of 20 MHz onward, ultrasound methods appear to be suitable for the identification of dermal atrophy [2, 18–20]. The disadvantages of the method are the following: it is time-consuming, the equipment is expensive and ultrasound scanners exceeding the 20-MHz range are as yet available only as a prototype [21]. Transepidermal water loss can be measured using an evaporimeter. This instrument detects effects of the corticosteroid on the stratum corneum, since it is the horny layer which represents the principal barrier to water loss [18].

In our own practice, in the framework of the long-term study of the topical application of corticosteroids to the volar forearm, we experimented with the early dectection of adverse effects by the method of skin surface microscopy. To this end we performed a hemilateral double-blind study with two corticosteroids of potency class III [6], BMV and PC, in an oil-in-water emulsion base. Like the findings in an earlier study [8], in which clobetasol 17-propionate was compared to hydrocortisone 17-butyrate, the cutaneous signs observed in the present investigations followed a reproducible, chronologically differentiated course, which in the case of BMV was as follows (fig. 3): slight distortion into parallel striae after an average of 16 days (IA); desquamation of the stratum corneum after 53 days (II); marked distortion into parallel striae after 67 days (IB); telangiectasias after 108 days (III); petechiae after 171 days (IV); ostiofollicular inflammation after 111 days (VI), and partial destruction of skin topography after 180 days (V). The course in the PC-treated skin was as follows (fig. 3): slight distortion into parallel striae after an average of 28 days (IA); desquamation of the stratum corneum after 91 days (II); marked distortion into parallel striae after an average of 89 days (IB), and telangiectasias after 54 days (III). No petechiae, ostiofollicular inflammation or destruction of the skin surface were observed.

If we compare the present results with the data from the hemilateral study of clobetasol 17-propionate (a highly potent group IV corticosteroid) and hydrocortisone 17-butyrate (a weak group II corticosteroid) [8], BMV and PC can be interpolated between these two substances in the hierarchy for time of onset of adverse effects.

In comparative ultrasound studies (20 MHz) with application of PC cream for 3 weeks, two groups of investigators working independently [22, 23] observed only a slight decrease in the thickness of the skin. Although the results of less recent studies [24] contradict these findings, these former studies were based on measurements made with early ultrasound equipment without B-mode images and show methodological errors in that white petrolatum (cutaneous edematization, which inhibits transepidermal water loss) or an untreated skin area served as a control instead of the corresponding cream base. In our own study, even with the use of the cream base, slight distortion in the form of parallel striae occurred due to loss of turgor, a finding which could only be attributed to the physicochemical properties of the vehicle.

Research on human skin fibroblast cultures has shown that, unlike the halogenated steroids clobetasol 17-propionate and BMV, corticosteroids esterified at positions 17 and 21 only slightly impair fibroblast synthesis of DNA, protein and collagen [25–27]. A lower cutaneous permeation rate of PC [28] as compared with other potent topical halogenated corticosteroids and rapid epidermal metabolization of the mother substance to the inactive 17,20,21-trihydroxysteroid [29] eliminate the correlation between effect and side effect [30]. Under occlusion or by using aluminum Finn chambers a physiological epidermal metabolism of PC cannot be expected. Thus, the results of Maas-Irslinger and Breitbart [31] which were seen under 22 h/day occlusion of 80% of the integument are practically irrelevant.

In conclusion, when applied reflecting clinical conditions the good risk/benefit ratio of PC was confirmed in the present double-blind study.

References

1 Christophers E, Schöpf E, Kligman AM, Stoughton RB: Topical Corticosteroid Therapy. A Novel Approach to Safer Drugs. New York, Raven Press, 1988.
2 Behrendt H, Korting HC: Klinische Prüfung von erwünschten und unerwünschten Wirkungen topisch applizierbarer Glukokortikosteroide am Menschen. Hautarzt 1990;41:2–8.
3 Braun Falco O, Sönnichsen N: Prednicarbat. Leitsubstanz fortschrittlicher Ekzemtherapie. Frankfurt, Universimed, 1991.
4 Stoughton RB, Cornell RC: Topical corticosteroids in dermatology; in Christophers E, Schöpf E, Kligman AM, Stoughton RB (eds): Topical Corticosteroid Therapy. New York, Raven Press, 1988, pp 1–12.
5 Bahmer A, Rohrer C: Ein Beitrag zur Abgrenzung früher Melanome mittels einer einfachen Methode der hochauflösenden Hautoberflächen-Fotografie. Akt Dermatol 1985;11:149–153.
6 Niedner R: Klassifikation der Glucocorticoide und ihre experimentelle Bewertung. Extracta Dermatol 1987;(suppl 1):11–15.
7 Feldmann RJ, Maibach HI: Percutaneous penetration of steroids in man. J Invest Dermatol 1969; 52:89–94.
8 Schulz H: Früherkennung kortikosteroidbedingter epidermaler Veränderungen mit der Methode der hochauflösenden Hautoberflächen-Fotografie. Therapiewoche 1988;38:2254–2260.
9 Marks R, Dykes P, Tan CY: Die Aufklärung und Messung kortikosteroidbedingter Atrophie der Haut. Akt Dermatol 1980;6:43–49.
10 Frosch PJ, Behrenbeck EM, Frosch K, Macher E: The Duhring chamber assay for corticosteroid atrophy. Br J Dermatol 1981;104:57–65.
11 Wendt H, Frosch PJ: Klinisch-pharmakologische Modelle zur Prüfung von Corticoidexterna. Basel, Karger, 1982.
12 Frosch PJ, Wendt H: Human models for quantification of corticosteroid adverse effects; in Maibach HI, Lowe NJ (eds): Models in Dermatology. Basel, Karger, 1985, vol 2, pp 5–15.
13 Frosch PJ, Wendt H, Kligman AM: Evaluation of corticosteroid atrophy by ammonium-hydroxide-blister-model. Arch Dermatol Res 1978;261:108.
14 Frosch PJ, Reckers R, Wendt H: The corticosteroid stratum corneum assay – A new bioassay to evaluate the risk of topical corticosteroids. Arch Dermatol Res 1981;270:252.
15 Dykes PJ, Marks R: Measurement of skin thickness: A comparison of two in vivo techniques with a conventional histometric method. J Invest Dermatol 1977;69:272–278.
16 Lubach D, Koppe R: Die kombinierte Kompressions- und Dickenmessung (K-D-Messung) einer Hautfalte. Ärztl Kosmetol 1984;14:243–252.
17 Lubach D, Hinz E: Untersuchungen über Entstehung und Rückbildung der dermalen Kortikosteroid-Atrophie. 1. Mitt.: Änderung der Hautfaltendicke. Dermatosen 1986;34:146–149.
18 Niedner R, Johannböcke R: Ausgewählte humanpharmakologische Modelle zur Untersuchung topischer Glukokortikoide. TW Dermatol 1991;21:298–306.
19 Breitbart EW, Hicks R, Kimmig W, Brockmann W, Mohr P: Ultraschall in der Dermatologie. Kreuzlingen, Derm A-Med, 1992.
20 Marks R: Survey of methods for assessment of corticosteroid atrophogenicity; in Christophers E, Schöpf E, Kligman AM, Stoughton RB (eds): Topical Corticosteroid Therapy. New York, Raven Press, 1988, pp 105–110.
21 Altmeyer P, Gammal S, Hoffmann K: Blick in die Haut – Ohne Schnitt und Biopsie. Münch Med Wochenschr 1990;18:14–22.

22 Korting HC, Vieluf D, Kerscher M: 0.25% prednicarbate cream and the corresponding vehicle induce less skin atrophy than 0.1% betamethasone-17-valerate cream and 0.05% clobetasol-17-propionate cream. Eur J Clin Pharmacol 1992;42:159–161.

23 Dykes PJ, Hill S, Marks R: Assessment of the atrophogenicity potential of corticosteroids by ultrasound and by epidermal biopsy under occlusive and nonocclusive conditions; in Christophers E, Schöpf E, Kligman AM, Stoughton RB (eds): Topical Corticosteroid Therapy. New York, Raven Press, 1988, pp 111–118.

24 Lubach D, Grüter H: Vergleichende Untersuchungen über die hautverdünnende Wirkung von Amcinonid und Prednicarbat an unterschiedlichen Körperregionen des Menschen. Akt Dermatol 1988;14:197–200.

25 Hein R, Krieg T: Wirkungen von Kortikoiden auf menschliche Fibroblasten in vitro. Z Hautkr 1991;66(suppl 5):13–17.

26 Gerbert G: Externe Kortikosteroidtherapie. Ärztl Kosmetol 1989;19:101–104.

27 Bernd A, Holzmann H: Zur Erfassung unerwünschter Corticoidwirkungen in der Zellkultur. Hautnah Dermatologie 1989;5:4–8.

28 Kim KH, Henderson NL: Kinetische Untersuchungen zur Hautpermeation und Biotransformation von Prednicarbat. Z Hautkr 1991;66(suppl 5):9–12.

29 Stache U, Alpermann HG: Zur Chemie und Pharmakologie des Prednicarbat (HOE 777), einem halogenfreien, topisch antiinflammatorisch wirksamen Derivat des Prednisolon-17-ethyl-Kohlensäureesters. Z Hautkr 1986;61(suppl 1):3–6.

30 Bodor N: The application of soft drug approaches to the design of safer corticosteroids; in Christophers E, Schöpf E, Kligman AM, Stoughton RB (eds): Topical Corticosteroid Therapy. New York, Raven Press, 1988, pp 13–25.

31 Maas-Irslinger R, Breitbart EW: Vergleichende Untersuchungen der systemischen und lokalen Nebenwirkungen von Prednicarbat und herkömmlichen, halogenierten Kortikosteroiden; in Macher E, Kolde G, Bröcker EB (eds): Jahrbuch der Dermatologie 1989/90. Zülpich, Biermann, 1990, pp 123–129.

H. Schulz, MD, Louise-Schröder-Strasse 20, D–59192 Bergkamen (FRG)

Korting HC, Maibach HI (eds): Topical Glucocorticoids with Increased Benefit/Risk Ratio.
Curr Probl Dermatol. Basel, Karger, 1993, vol 21, pp 140–146

....

Influence of Glucocorticoid Substances and the Vehicle on Skin Irritancy: Determination by Profilometry

Hans Christian Korting

Dermatologische Klinik und Poliklinik (Direktor: Prof. Dr. *G. Plewig*) der
Ludwig-Maximilians-Universität München, BRD

Xerosis or dry skin is the most frequent individual characteristic of atopic eczema, the most important indication for topical glucocorticoid use. This type of state of the skin is clinically characterized by brittleness and predisposition to fine fissures [1]. While dry skin can by principle also be found in about a quarter of the normal population, it is found in patients suffering from atopic dermatitis in more than 90% [2]. An état craquélé representing an aggravated stage of atopic dry skin, however, does not only represent an indication for topical glucocorticoids but can also be the consequence of topical glucocorticoid treatment as shown by Björnberg [3]. In fact, this investigator was able to provoke 'erythema craquélé' on normal skin by applying a glucocorticoid. This certainly is a major concern as an unwanted effect of topical glucocorticoids of this appearance might lead to prolonged therapy in patients initially suffering from atopic eczema. Such an unwanted effect by principle can go back to the action of the so-called active ingredient, in the given context the topical glucocorticoid, or the vehicle. In fact, side effects due to vehicle action seemingly are not rare. Even in the context of well-controlled comparative clinical trials, such effects are fairly frequently seen, i.e., in several percent of patients. According to the series of trials analyzed globally by Akers [4], adverse events due to vehicles are even more frequent than those due to the glucocorticoids proper: while in a subgroup of 343 patients receiving a vehicle preparation side effects were noted in 6.7%, this was only the case in 4.39% of 5,698 exposures to glucocorticoid treatment. In the former group of patients, irritation (3.8%), pruritus (1.2%) and dryness (0.6%) were most prominent. About the same was true of the latter group, irritation, itching, burning and stinging, dryness and scaling being found in 1.30, 0.95, 0.81, 0.46 and 0.30% respectively. But not only in patients on vehicles was the influence of the dosage form evident: in fact, gel preparations caused more often adverse events, in particular pruritus and dryness, than cream and ointment preparations, the figures reading 9.4, 2.8 and 1.5% respectively. This influence of the type of vehicle even seemed more marked than the influence of the type of glucocorticoid. However, more potent glucocorticoid preparations were linked to unwanted effects slightly more often than less potent ones.

To get more insight into the relative influence of various glucocorticoid compounds and the composition of the vehicle on the surface structure of normal human skin, skin roughness as one prominent parameter of dry skin was addressed parallel to the clinical appearance of the skin in one orienting and one full-size trial. Skin roughness, as expressed by the so-called mean peak-to-valley height, has been demonstrated to represent a valid parameter in the context of eczema and its treatment by anti-inflammatory agents [5].

Materials and Methods

This is a report on additional investigations in the context of two double-blind controlled trials in normal human beings performed primarily to address the influence of various glucocorticoid and base preparations on skin thickness as to be measured by ultrasound. With the first trial, 6 out of 24 individuals were in addition checked for skin surface roughness to get orienting data on the influence of a commercial oil-in-water emulsion and the addition of a nonhalogenated double ester-type glucocorticoid to this base. In the second trial, 12 individuals out of 24 were additionally analyzed to address the influence of a conventional medium potent and highly potent glucocorticoid in dependence on the vehicle: cream vs. ointment.

In the first trial the four treaments were as follows: (A) prednicarbate 0.25% cream; (B) the vehicle of prednicarbate 0.25% cream; (C) betamethasone-17-valerate 0.1% cream, and (D) clobetasol-17-propionate 0.05% cream.

In the second trial the following four treatments were applied: (A) triamcinolone acetonide 0.1% cream; (B) triamcinolone acetonide 0.1% ointment; (C) clobetasol-17-propionate 0.05% cream, and (D) clobetasol-17-propionate 0.05% ointment.

In trial 1, either preparation A or B was applied to one forearm and preparation C or D to the other corresponding to a randomized blocks design. In the second trial, allocation of the treatment modalities also was at random. At each point of time, 0.1–0.2 ml of each preparation was applied to the proximal part of the volar side of the forearm close to the elbow. The area itself consisted of 4 × 4 cm. During the investigation this open application took place once in the morning and once in the evening over a period of 6 weeks.

In the first trial, visual inspection took place on days 0, 4, 7, 14, 21, 28, 35, 42 and 63, focussing on the manifestation of eczema craquélé defined by dry, scaly skin with reticulate fissures [6].

In the second trial on the corresponding days, visual inspection was directed at the following score: 0 = no clinical changes, normal skin; 1 = erythema craquélé; 2 = teleangiectasia, and 3 = striae distensae.

Table 1. Clinical changes due to the application of various glucocorticoid preparations over time

Preparation:	A			B			C			D		
Day:	0	21	42	0	21	42	0	21	42	0	21	42
Erythema	–	2	3	–	–	2	–	4	7	–	3	6
Eczema craquélé	–	–	–	–	–	–	–	5	5	–	–	–
Teleangiectasia	–	–	–	–	–	–	–	1	2	–	–	–
Stria distensae	–	–	–	–	–	–	–	–	–	–	–	–

Preparations: A = triamcinolone acetonide cream; B = triamcinolone acetonide ointment; C = clobetasol-17-propionate cream; D = clobetasol-17-propionate ointment.

While in the first trial profilometry was only performed on days 0 and 42 (i.e., before and after treatment) this was the case on days 0, 21, 42 and 63 in the second trial. While in the first trial only 6 individuals were included, the corresponding figure in the second one amounted to 12 representing a fully balanced subpopulation. The procedure used to analyze the skin surface profile is described elsewhere in more detail [7]. In brief, replicas of the skin surface treated were obtained using dental silicone rubber impression material (Silasoft N, Detax, Karlsruhe, FRG). These replicas were scanned at six different angles with the Hommel tester T 2000 (Hommel, Villingen-Schwenningen, FRG). Among the various parameters of the roughness defined by German industrial standards (DIN 4768 and DIN 4762) the mean peak-to-valley height RZ_{DIN} was chosen for final evaluation.

While the data in the first trial were only analyzed descriptively, in the second trial Wilcoxon's test for unpaired samples was used for the comparison of the four treatment groups and Spearman's test for correlation studies. $p < 0.05$ was considered to indicate a difference [for further details of both trials, cf. 8, 9].

Results

In the first trial, out of the 6 volunteers investigated for skin surface roughness, 4 received betamethasone-17-valerate 0.1% cream, 3 prednicarbate 0.25% cream, 3 the corresponding vehicle, 2 clobetasol-17-propionate 0.05% cream. In the latter 2 individuals, overt eczema craquélé was seen which made precocious discontinuation of treatment inevitable. Therefore, skin roughness could not be addressed by profilometry at the end of the scheduled 6-week application period. The mean RZ_{DIN} values for the three other types of treatment are given in figure 1.

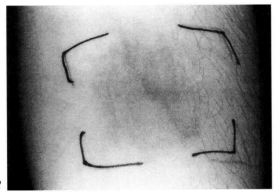

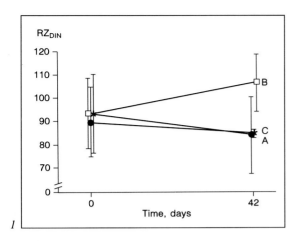

Fig. 1. Skin surface roughness as determined by profilometry addressing the RZ_{DIN} value before and after 6-week application of prednicarbate 0.25% cream (A), the corresponding vehicle (B) and betamethasone-17-valerate 0.1% cream (C). [From 8, with permission.]

Fig. 2. Eczema craquélé after 3 weeks' twice daily open application of clobetasol-17-propionate 0.05% cream to the proximal flexor part of the forearm. [From 9, with permission.]

In the second trial the typical clinical picture of eczema craquélé was seen in 5 volunteers in 12, to an extent making discontinuation of treatment inevitable. The clinical aspect is demonstrated in figure 2. Data on the various possible unwanted effects addressed visually with the various preparations over time are given in table 1. From day 14 onward the score for eczema craquélé characterized

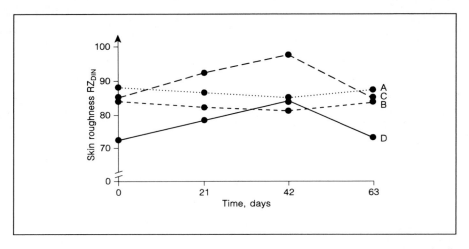

Fig. 3. RZ$_{DIN}$ values representing skin surface roughness before and under application of various glucocorticoid preparations as well as after discontinuation (A = triamcinolone acetonide 0.1% ointment; B = triamcinolone acetonide 0.1% cream; C = clobetasol-17-propionate 0.05% ointment; D = clobetasol-17-propionate 0.05% cream). [From 9, with permission.]

by dilated vessels and skin surface cracks was markedly higher with both preparations containing clobetasol-17-propionate as compared to the ones containing triamcinolone acetonide ($p < 0.05$). In general, skin exposed to a cream form tended to be more prone to overt changes.

The mean RZ$_{DIN}$ representing skin surface roughness before, under and after application of the various drugs is shown in figure 3. While there was no major increase in roughness with both forms incorporating triamcinolone acetonide, this was the case with both corresponding forms containing clobetasol-17-propionate. Among the latter two the cream form increased skin surface roughness more ($p < 0.05$).

Discussion

In the first trial, a cream base representing an oil-in-water emulsion increased skin surface roughness which was not the case when 0.25% prednicarbate was added. This implies that by principle cream bases considered for topical application of glucocorticoids can influence the state of the skin surface. Although visible effects were not seen, this backs the hypothesis to be derived from the data by

Akers [4] that vehicles may contribute a lot to the minor unwanted effects seen upon the open application of topical glucocorticoid preparations. Recently, Van der Valk and Maibach [10] have been able to demonstrate that several topical glucocorticoids are not able to suppress irritant skin reaction due to sodium lauryl sulfate solution. Recently, we have in addition demonstrated that this also applies to prednicarbate [11]. Thus, skin irritation due to an oil-in-water emulsion might be remarkably different from the one induced by the well-known model irritant sodium lauryl sulfate. Under clinical aspects it is fortunate to see that prednicarbate 0.25% cream does not influence skin surface roughness negatively.

According to the results of the second trial this also applies to triamcinolone acetonide in both usual vehicles, i.e., the base cream and ointment at the usual concentration of 0.1%. With clobetasol-17-propionate 0.05% this is clearly different. Here both forms increase skin surface roughness. Yet it is remarkable that this applies to the cream form even more than to the ointment form. This finding is further corroborated by the results of clinical inspection: in general, visible unwanted effects are rather linked to the cream form, and unwanted effects exceeding erythema are even exclusively seen with the cream form. As both corresponding base preparations were not tested it can at the moment not be decided definitely if the glucocorticoid or the vehicle is causative. Yet it is tempting to speculate that it is at least to a remarkable portion the glucocorticoid compound by itself which induces skin rougness, as corresponding clinical signs have so far never been linked to a base preparation of the water-in-oil-emulsion type. This in other terms means that there is a dissociation between unwanted effects on the epidermal and dermal level with the medium potent glucocorticoid triamcinolone acetonide and the highly potent congener clobetasol-17-propionate. While both reduce skin thickness markedly after a few weeks' time [12], only clobetasol-17-propionate also influences the skin surface, i.e., the epidermis negatively.

In clinical practice, according to the present findings, increased skin surface roughness or even eczema craquelé need not be feared with the repeated open application of both new and conventional medium potent topical glucocorticoids. With a highly potent one, however, one has to be afraid that clinical signs originally indicative of atopic eczema representing a prime indication for topical glucocorticoids as drugs of first choice might later represent unwanted effects of the drug used.

As profilometry can detect unwanted effects on the skin surface structure before visible changes turn up, this modern bioengineering method should be included into the armamentarium of the clinical dermatopharmacologist when it comes to the evaluation of new glucocorticoid preparations. It looks particularly helpful to interpret data thus obtained before the background of parallel data on skin thickness is obtained by ultrasound analysis.

Acknowledgments

I am grateful to Dr. Th. Höhler and K. Wörz, Cassella-Riedel Pharma GmbH, Frankfurt, FRG, as well as Dr. K. Schnitker from Bielefeld, FRG, for providing the test preparations and for statistical analysis.

References

1   Hanifin JM: Atopic dermatitis; in Marks R (ed): Eczema. London, Dunitz, 1992, pp 77–101.
2   Diepgen TL, Fartasch M: Recent epidemiological and genetic studies in atopic dermatitis; in Rajka G (ed): International Symposium on Atopic Dermatitis. Acta Derm Venereol (Stockh) 1992(suppl 176):13–18.
3   Björnberg A: Erythema craquélé provoked by corticosteroids on normal skin. Acta Derm Venereol (Stockh) 1982;62:147–151.
4   Akers WM: Risks of unoccluded topical steroids in clinical trials. Arch Dermatol 1980;116:786–788.
5   Nissen HP, Biltz H, Kreysel HW: Profilometrie, eine Methode zur Beurteilung der therapeutischen Wirksamkeit von Kamillosan-Salbe. Z Hautkr 1988;63:184–190.
6   Smolle J, Juettner F-M, Kerl H: Exsikkationsekzematoide. Pathogenese, Differentialdiagnose, Therapie. Ärztl Kosmetol 1986;16:184–189.
7   Vieluf D: Skin roughness-measuring methods and dependence on washing procedure; in Braun-Falco O, Korting HC (eds): Skin Cleansing with Synthetic Detergents. Chemical, Ecological and Clinical Aspects. Berlin, Springer, 1992, pp 116–129.
8   Korting HC, Kerscher M, Vieluf D, Mehringer L, Megele M, Braun-Falco O: Commercial glucocorticoid formulations and skin dryness. Could it be caused by the vehicle? Acta Derm Venereol (Stockh) 1991;71:261–263.
9   Kerscher MJ, Korting HC, Mehringer L, Mätzig R: 0.05% clobetasol-17-propionate cream and ointment but not the corresponding 0.1% triamcinolone acetonide preparations increase skin surface roughness: Hints at a possible dissociation of unwanted epidermal and dermal effecs. Skin Pharmacol, in press.
10 Van der Valk P, Maibach HI: Do topical corticosteroids modulate skin irritation in human beings? Assessments by transepidermal water loss and visual scoring. J Am Acad Dermatol 1989;21:519–522.
11 Schäfer-Korting M, Korting HC, Kerscher MJ, Lenhart S: Prednicarbate activity and benefit/risk ratio in relation to other topical glucocorticoids. Clin Pharmacol Ther, in press.
12 Kerscher MJ, Korting HC: Comparative atrophogenicity potential of medium and highly potent topical glucocorticoids in cream and ointment according to ultrasound analysis. Skin Pharmacol 1992;5:77–80.

Prof. Hans C. Korting, MD, Dermatologische Klinik und Poliklinik der
Ludwig-Maximilians-Universität, Frauenlobstrasse 9–11, D–80337 München (FRG)

Korting HC, Maibach HI (eds): Topical Glucocorticoids with Increased Benefit/Risk Ratio.
Curr Probl Dermatol. Basel, Karger, 1993, vol 21, pp 147–156

....

Prednicarbate after Different Forms of Administration

Plasma Levels of Drug and Metabolites and Effects on Endogenous Cortisol Levels in Humans

J. Barth[a], *G. Hochhaus*[b], *H. Derendorf*[b], *K.H. Lehr*[c], *Th. Höhler*[d], *H. Moellmann*[a]

[a] Medizinische Universitätsklinik und Poliklinik «Bergmannsheil» der Ruhruniversität Bochum, BRD;
[b] College of Pharmacy, University of Florida, Gainesville, Fla., USA;
[c] Radiochemisches Labor, Hoechst AG, Frankfurt/Hoechst, BRD;
[d] Cassella-Riedel Pharma GmbH, Frankfurt/Main, BRD

In the last decade, novel approaches in the field of topical glucocorticoids attempted to provide drugs which induce the desired topical effects without undesired systemic side effects. Thus, compounds have been designed with high local activity which are efficiently metabolized once they have entered the systemic circulation.

Prednicarbate, the C_{17}-ethylcarbonate C_{21}-propionate double ester of prednisolone (fig. 1), represents a new glucocorticoid prodrug for topical use which was selected on the basis of rapid enzymatic degradation. According to animal studies, it is efficiently cleaved in the skin, to yield the prednisolone 17-ester (fig. 1). This species is the pharmacologically active compound with a receptor-binding affinity comparable to that of dexamethasone [1]. Upon absorption into the systemic circulation, it is thought to be further metabolized to the less active prednisolone. The high activity of the prednisolone 17-ethylcarbonate and the rapid inactivation are responsible for its distinct topical effects without pronounced systemic side effects.

Because of the above characteristics, prednicarbate was successfully introduced for dermatological use. However, the same properties are also highly desirable for other types of topical administration, such as via the pulmonary or ocular

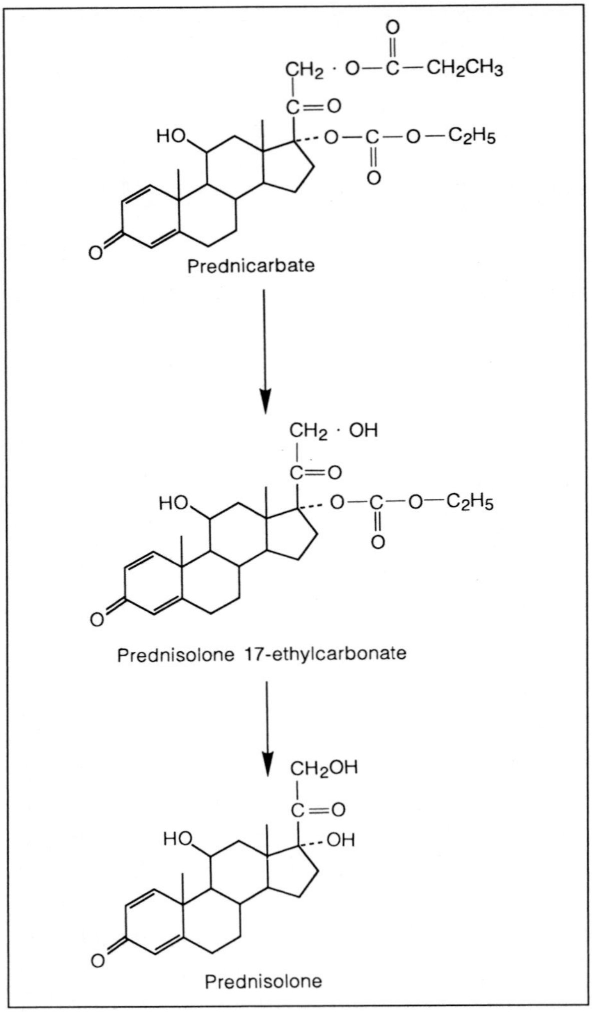

Fig. 1. Potential metabolic route of prednicarbate.

route. In order to evaluate its general suitability for local delivery, we extend a previous report to the pharmacokinetic profile of prednicarbate [2] by comparing drug profiles after pulmonary application (inhalation and intrabronchial instillation), after dermal administration and, for control purposes, after oral delivery in humans.

Materials and Methods

Study Design

This crossover controlled study was performed in 8 healthy volunteers (average age 30.8 years) who abstained from any medication for a period of 4 weeks prior to the study and from caffeine, alcohol and nicotine during the study day. A washout period of at least 1 week was allowed between the treatments. The study was approved by the internal review board of the University of Bochum. Only 3 volunteers received intrabronchial instillation of prednicarbate.

Cutaneous Administration. 75 mg of prednicarbate in 0.25% emollient ointment (water-in-oil emulsion, ointment base: octyldocanole, glycerol ester, white vaseline, edetic acid, magnesium sulfate and water) was applied thinly to the trunk and upper arms, representing about 50% of the total body surface and allowed to stay under occlusion for 12 h.

Oral Delivery. 40 mg of prednicarbate was suspended in 10 ml of water and administered to the volunteers with a total of 100 ml of water.

Pulmonary Delivery via Inhalation. 4 ml of crystal suspension (40 mg of prednicarbate) was diluted with 4 ml of saline. The drug was inhaled with a clinically used nebulizer (Pariboy, Paul Ritzau, Pari-Werk GmbH, Starnberg, FRG) under deep breathing over a period of 60–70 min.

Intrabronchial Instillation. 3 volunteers received a direct intrabronchial instillation of 40 mg of prednicarbate. After anesthesia of the throat and the nasal membranes, a flexible bronchoscope (Olympus, Hamburg, FRG) was introduced into the central bronchial system. Using the working channel of the bronchoscope a thin plastic catheter was introduced into a subsegment of the 4th or 5th lung segment. Directly after the dose was sprayed into the lung segment, bronchoscope and catheter were removed.

Controls. Blood samples were taken in a treatment-free period of 10 h for the determination of a control cortisol secretion profile.

Blood Sampling. 8 ml of blood were collected before application of the drug and 5, 15, 30, 45, 60, 90, 120, 150, 180, 240, 360, 480, 600, 720 and 1,440 min after start of the treatment. After addition of 800 μl of an esterase inhibitor cocktail (12 g NaF in 100 ml of isotonic saline), the blood was centrifuged for 10 min at 4 °C and the plasma was immediately frozen and stored at –20 °C.

Corticosteroid Analysis

After the addition of dexamethasone as internal standard, 1 ml of plasma was extracted with 5 ml of butyl tertiary methyl ester.

Prednicarbate, prednisolone C_{17}-ethylcarbonate, prednisolone and cortisol levels were determined by a reverse-phase HPLC method using a C_{18}-Zorbax® column. A stepwise gradient was performed with a tetrahydrofurane (A)-H_2O (B) mixture as mobile phase (step 1: 0–9 min, 85% A; step 2: 9–17 min, 45% A). The detection limit for prednicarbate, prednisolone 17-ethylcarbonate, prednisolone and hydrocortisone was 10, 20, 10 and 5 ng/ml, respectively.

Pharmacokinetic Analysis

Data on prednicarbate, prednisolone 17-ethylcarbonate and prednisolone were evaluated by compartmental and noncompartmental analysis. AUC, mean residence time and bioavailability were determined by standard noncompartmental approaches. Compartmental analysis was performed using the nonlinear curve fitting procedure MINSQ under the assumption that all prednicarbate is transformed into 17-ethylcarbonate, which is consequently fully converted into prednisolone. Data published for prednisolone were incorporated into the model whenever possible [3]. Fits for all treatment groups were done simultaneously. Statistical evaluation of the pharmacodynamic data (hydrocortisone suppression) was performed with the areas under the effect/time curves as cumulative parameter using the statistical package SAS.

Results

After percutaneous administration of 75 mg prednicarbate, neither the intact drug nor the metabolites prednisolone 17-ethylcarbonate and prednisolone could be detected in the plasma of the volunteers at any of the investigated time points.

After intrabronchial instillation, inhalation and oral delivery, prednisolone 17-ethylcarbonate and prednisolone but no intact prednicarbate were detectable in the plasma.

Time profiles of plasma levels are shown in figures 2–4. Resulting pharmacokinetic parameters are listed in table 1. The half-life of prednisolone 17-ethylcarbonate was 1.6 h. The mean residence times for prednisolone 17-ethylcarbonate and prednisolone were between 3.1 and 5.9 h, respectively. The biovailability calculated from plasma prednisolone levels under the assumption that the entire prednicarbate is converted into prednisolone was similar for the oral and instillation route (14 ± 7 and $15 \pm 4\%$, respectively), while a lower value was observed for the inhalation data ($5 \pm 2\%$).

Plasma hydrocortisone levels after the various treatments (fig. 5, 6) directly reflected the amount of drug absorbed (fig. 7). Thus, cumulative cortisol levels in the nontreatment phase (451 ± 329 ng/ml·h) and after percutaneous administration (412 ng/ml·h) and inhalation (403 ± 671 ng/ml·h) were not significantly different for the 10-hour observation period. A significant suppression was observed after oral administration (976 ± 351 ng/ml·h) and intrabronchial instillation (858 ± 290 ng/ml·h). A similar picture was observed for the 24-hour obser-

Fig. 2. Concentration-time curve of prednisolone 17-ethylcarbonate (△) and prednisolone (▲) after oral administration.

Fig. 3. Concentration-time curve of prednisolone 17-ethylcarbonate (△) and prednisolone (▲) after pulmonary instillation.

Fig. 4. Concentration-time curve of prednisolone 17-ethylcarbonate (△) and prednisolone (▲) after inhalation.

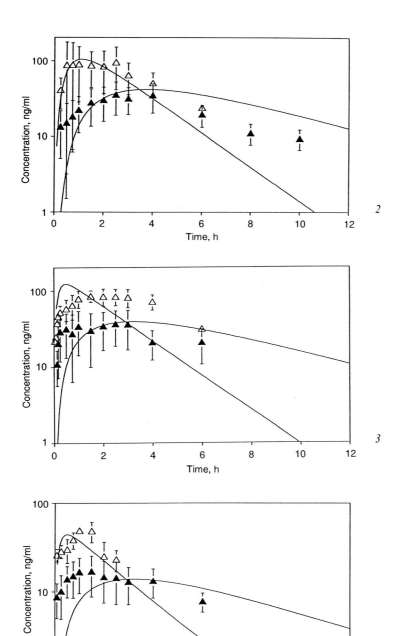

2

3

4

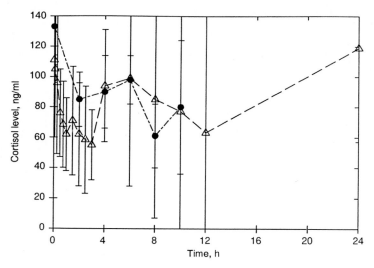

Fig. 5. Endogenous cortisol levels after control (●) and percutaneous administration (△).

Table 1. Pharmacokinetic data after inhalation, instillation and oral delivery of 40 mg prednicarbate

Prednisolone 17-ethylcarbonate	Terminal half-life, h	1.6 ± 1
	Mean residence time, h	
	Inhalation	2.4 ± 0.2
	Intrabronchial	3.6 ± 0.4
	Oral	3.1 ± 0.6
Prednisolone	Terminal half-life, h	3.5^a
	Mean residence time, h	
	Inhalation	4.8 ± 0.7
	Intrabronchial	3.1 ± 0.4
	Oral	5.9 ± 0.6
Bioavailability[b], %	Oral	15 ± 4
	Instillation	14 ± 7
	Inhalation	8 ± 2

[a] Taken from the literature.
[b] Area under the prednisolone/time curves were compared with those obtained from the literature after intravenous injection.

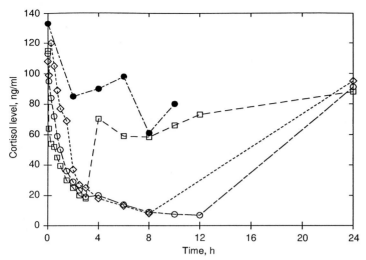

Fig. 6. Endogenous cortisol levels after control (●), inhalation (□), instillation (◊) and oral delivery (○). Standard deviations are not given for the reason of clarity.

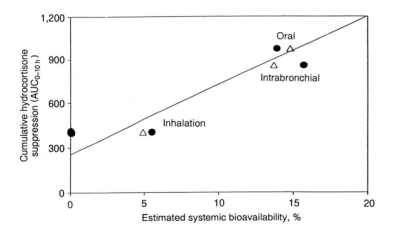

Fig. 7. Relationship between the area under the prednisolone concentration-time curve and the cortisol suppression. ● = Determined by noncompartmental analysis; △ = determined by compartmental analysis.

vation period. However, the cortisol suppression was not sustained after these forms of administration, as cortisol levels returned to normal after 24 h (fig. 5, 6).

Discussion

Prednicarbate has been introduced as topical glucocorticoid with the goal of inducing distinct local effects with the avoidance of systemic side effects. A lipophilic diester concept was followed to ensure sufficient lipophilicity for percutaneous absorption. Prednicarbate does not bind to the glucocorticoid receptor and is thus a glucocorticoid prodrug. It needs to be cleaved to the pharmacologically active prednisolone 17-ethylcarbonate, a drug with a receptor-binding affinity comparable to that of dexamethasone [1]. Our studies after oral and pulmonary administration have clearly shown that prednicarbate is efficiently metabolized, and the appearance of significant amounts of prednisolone 17-ethylcarbonate demonstrated the validity of the drug design concept for nondermal application. It also supports previous reports on the efficient metabolism of prednicarbate in in vitro systems [4]. Plasma level/time profiles after pulmonary application revealed the principal suitability of this compound in asthma therapy, as the prodrug is efficiently cleaved to generate the pharmacologically active drug. This is subsequently efficiently eliminated to reduce systemic side effects. Additional studies, however, have to demonstrate that the activation step is located in the bronchopulmonary system, since this is a requirement for site-specific topical application. The plasma concentration profiles after oral delivery and instillation were very similar, in sharp contrast to previous findings for methylprednisolone and triamcinolone acetonide solutions [5]. This might indicate that the rate-limiting step for the absorption rate is the dissolution of the glucocorticoid crystal suspensions.

In addition, the relatively short half-life of prednisolone 17-ethylcarbonate backs the concept of efficient deactivation of prednisolone 17-ethylcarbonate, and indeed the elimination of prednicarbate is comparable with that of other fast-eliminating glucocorticoids such as triamcinolone acetonide [6] or budesonide [7].

The lack of prednicarbate metabolites in plasma after percutaneous administration is in agreement with the low biovailability of prednicarbate found in animal models (2–6%) [8]. Thus, more detailed studies employing either ultrasensitive analytical tools for plasma determinations or the determination of urine excretion profiles should be performed to quantify the dermal absorption pattern.

Interestingly, the bioavailability based upon prednisolone equivalents was also low after oral delivery, inhalation and instillation. While the very low bioavailability after inhalation confirms the often reported drug loss within the inhalation procedure, results for the oral and instillation routes were rather surprising, as both administration routes generally result in higher systemic bioavailabilities for glucocorticoids [5]. We, therefore, speculate that the proposed metabolic route – a full conversion from prednicarbate to prednisolone – has to be reevaluated. Our data argue against the unidirectional metabolic fate of prednicarbate, and for a multidirectional metabolic inactivation of prednicarbate and/or prednisolone 17-ethylcarbonate through a variety of enzymatic pathways.

A distinct cortisol suppression was seen after inhalation, instillation or oral delivery. Our data pool was also able to show a direct relationship between the degree of cortisol depression and the area under the prednisolone time curves as indicator of the systemic spillover of topically applied drug. This suppression was, however, fully reversible after 24 h, contrary to systemically active drugs such as dexamethasone [9]. This argues for the suitability of prednicarbate for pulmonary delivery, particularly as the necessary doses for pulmonary prednicarbate delivery will be far below those employed in this study. Dermal application of prednicarbate did not affect the circulating cortisol levels, supporting previous reports in children and adult volunteers and patients [10, 11].

In summary, after dermal administration, drug-related plasma levels are too small to induce any effects on the hypothalamic-pituitary-adrenal axis. Preliminary results after inhalation are promising, and the clinical evaluation of prednicarbate in pulmonary diseases might be considered.

References

1   Poertner M, Moellmann H, Rohdewald P: Glucocorticoid receptors in human synovial tissue and relative receptor affinities of glucocorticoid-21-esters. Pharmacol Res 1988;5:623–627.
2   Barth J, Lehr KH, Derendorf H, Moellmann HW, Hoehler T, Hochhaus G: Studies on the pharmacokinetics and metabolism of prednicarbate after cutaneous and oral administration. Skin Pharmacol, in press.
3   Derendorf H, Rohdewald P, Moellmann H, Rehder J, Barth J, Neveling D: Pharmacokinetics of prednisolone after high doses of prednisolone hemisuccinate. Biopharm Drug Dispos 1985;6:423–432.
4   Kim KH, Henderson NL: Kinetic studies of skin permeation and biotransformation of prednicarbate; in Christophers E (ed): Topical Corticosteroid Therapy: A Novel Approach to Safer Drugs. New York, Raven Press, 1988, pp 49–56.
5   Barth J, Möllmann A, Hochhaus G, Derendorf H, Möllmann HW: Absorption and transfer of water-soluble glucocorticoids through pulmonary membranes. Atemwegs-Lungenkr 1989;15:412–416.
6   Moellmann H, Rohdewald P, Schmidt EW, Salomon V, Derendorf H: Pharmacokinetics of triamcinolone acetonide and its phosphate ester. Eur J Pharmacol 1985;29:85–89.

7   Ryrfeld A, Toennesson M, Nilsson E, Wikby A: Pharmacokinetic studies of a potent glucocorticoid (budesonide) in dogs by high performance liquid chromatography. J Steroid Biochem 1978;10: 317–324.

8   Kellner H-M, Eckert HG, Fehlhaber HW, Hornke I, Oekonomopoulos R: Untersuchungen zur Pharmakokinetik und zur Biotransformation nach topischer Anwendung des lokalen Kortikoids Prednicarbat. Z Hautkr 1986;61:(suppl 1):18–40.

9   Loew D, Schuster O, Graul EH: Dose-dependent pharmacokinetics of dexamethasone. Eur J Clin Pharmacol 1986;30:225–230.

10 Schroepl F, Schubert C: Long term study on local steroids using the example of prednicarbate; in Christophers E (ed): Topical Corticosteroid Therapy: A Novel Approach to Safer Drugs. New York, Raven Press, 1988, pp 155–168.

11 Schroepl F: Plasma cortisol concentrations following whole-body application of Hoe 777 (predni-carbate); in Christophers E (ed): Topical Corticosteroid Therapy: A Novel Approach to Safer Drugs. New York, Raven Press, 1988, pp 169–180.

Günther Hochhaus, PhD, College of Pharmacy (Box J-494), University of Florida,
Gainesville, FL 32610 (USA)

Korting HC, Maibach HI (eds): Topical Glucocorticoids with Increased Benefit/Risk Ratio.
Curr Probl Dermatol. Basel, Karger, 1993, vol 21, pp 157–169

....

Clinical Efficacy of Topical Glucocorticoid Preparations and Other Types of Dermatics in Inflammatory Diseases, Particularly in Atopic Dermatitis

Roland Niedner, Erwin Schöpf

Universitäts-Hautklinik, Freiburg i.Br., BRD

The treatment of inflammatory skin diseases such as eczema, lichen planus, discoid lupus erythematosus, atopic dermatitis and others is not restricted to glucocorticosteroids. There are indeed a wide range of therapeutic possibilities, which are listed in table 1. This list is incomplete, as it does not take into account the so-called alternative methods such as acupuncture, *L*-peptides and ozone.

Subsequently, we will focus on four themes: (1) topical glucocorticosteroids (TCSs); (2) nonsteroidal anti-inflammatory drugs (NSAIDs), in particular bufexamac; (3) natural moisturizing factors (NMFs), in particular urea, and (4) high-dose ultraviolet A-1 (UVA-1) irradiation.

Topical Glucocorticosteroids

Fundamentally, the efficacy of TCSs is indisputable, but their strength depends on many factors (table 2). Cornell and Maibach published in 1992 [1] a list of skin diseases which are variably sensitive to TCSs (table 3). Although we cannot agree completely with their division, and though the list is incomplete, we must consider that the prototype of inflammatory skin diseases, i.e. the different types of eczema and in particular atopic dermatitis, will respond more or less to TCSs.

The inhibition of mitosis in the basal epidermal layer and dermal fibroblasts is an obligatory effect of potent TCSs. This fact is of significance in the treatment of psoriasis. Depending on the type of this disease, it may be sensitive, less sensi-

Table 1. Treatment of inflammatory skin diseases

Topical glucocorticoids	NSAIDs
Tar preparations	Dyes
Dithranol	Antiseptics
Mast cell blockers	Tannic acid
Natural moisturizing factors	Salicylic aid
Ointments bases	Bathing
Antibiotics	Antimycotics
Unsaturated fatty acids	Antihistamines
Ultraviolet radiation	X-rays
Immunomodulation	
Balneoheliotherapy	Climatotherapy
Hypoallergenic diet	Psychotherapy

Table 2. Factors on which efficacy of TCSs depends

Type of skin disease
Type of vehicle
Concentration of TCS
Penetration
   Depot
   Site of application
   Age of skin
   Damaged stratum corneum
   Occlusion
Potency ranking

tive or even resistant. But besides the type-dependent varying efficacy of corticosteroids, it must be considered that a reduction of the corticosteroid dosage or especially an interruption of therapy induces very often a relapse which is harder to treat and requires more and more potent types of TCSs to ameliorate the dermatitis [2]. Therefore, as standard therapy for psoriasis Germany dithranol is still used, leading to longer periods of disease-free skin, as well as PUVA irradiation.

Normally the inflammatory signs in the skin begin to fade within 3 or 4 days (atopic dermatitis), but it takes approximately 14 days and sometimes even longer (psoriasis) to obtain sufficient clearing. The basis for these differences is poorly

Table 3. Responsiveness of dermatoses to TCSs

TCS-resistant dermatoses
Plaque-type psoriasis
Palmoplantar psoriasis
Lichen simplex chronicus
Dyshidrotic eczema (chronic stage)
Lichen planus
Granuloma annulare
Necrobiosis lipoidica diabeticorum
Sarcoidosis

Moderately TCS-sensitive dermatoses
Psoriasis, non-plaque-type
Parapsoriasis
Atopic dermatitis – adults
Nummular eczema
Primary irritant dermatitis
Papular urticaria secondary to bites
Discoid lupus erythematosus

TCS-sensitive dermatoses
Psoriasis, intertriginous area
Atopic dermatitis – children
Seborrheic dermatitis
Sunburn
Intertrigo
Pruritus ani, vulvae, scroti
Pityriasis rosea (pruritus)

---

understood and cannot be explained by simple differences in drug penetration into the skin. It may be related to different inflammatory patterns present in both diseases [3].

The affinity between the TCS and the vehicle is a determining factor of the efficacy and penetration into the skin. The higher the degree of glucocorticosteroid saturation in the vehicle the greater is the therapeutic effect. Malzfeldt et al. [4] demonstrated that two preparations of betamethasone benzoate of the same concentration but with different vehicles had a different efficacy. On the other hand, Stoughton showed that the blanching effect of triamcinolone was nearly identical though the concentrations differed by a factor of 20. It may be that even the lowest concentration of 0.025% triamcinolone acetonide was already the maximum concentration required for binding to the receptors. Thus, it is explainable that the dilution of a glucocorticosteroid in certain ointment bases does not reduce its potency. That is why one should be cautious and not use glucocorticosteroid ointments without measuring their liberation and penetration of the glucocorticosteroid.

Besides the discussion about controversial indications for TCSs and besides the use in specific diseases, the clinical effectiveness depends on the type of TCS. For many years three generations of TCSs were known, but in recent years the very interesting fourth-generation corticosteroids were developed, the so-called soft steroids, i.e. hydrocortisone butyrate, hydrocortisone aceponate, hydrocortisone butyrate propionate and prednicarbate. Practically every functional group of the corticosteroid molecule has been modified in order to achieve a select effect. These derivatives, which are free from halogens, are esterified at position C-17 and/or C-21 and display relatively high anti-inflammatory but only weak antiproliferative effects. This dissociation of their efficacy profile leads to a greater safety in the treatmet with TCSs. Although a definitive separation of anti-inflammatory activity (efficacy) and atrophogenicity (toxicity) cannot be made to date, the tendency is going undoubtedly to the soft steroids. These can be defined as active drugs characterized by a controllable in vivo metabolism to nontoxic moieties after having developed their therapeutic effect. Because of their labile ester bonds the molecule will be degraded already within the skin (first-pass effect), minimizing systemic side effects. Therefore, the main objective of drug design should not be activity alone, but also the therapeutic index, i.e. the ratio of efficacy to toxicity [3].

All topical glucocorticoid brands available on the German market are grouped according to potency [6] in tables 4–7. The potency cannot be given as absolute values, because it depends on many factors such as the liberation of the TCS from its vehicle, the age of the skin and the type of dermatosis.

In order to obtain the optimal clinical efficacy of TCSs, some general rules have to be considered. In inflammatory skin diseases, such as acute exacerbation of atopic dermatitis, TCS treatment has to begin with the most potent steroid. Schalla [7] discussed the possibility of applying initially rather low potent steroids such as hydrocortisone esters because the barrier function of the epidermis may be disturbed in the acute inflammatory phase of atopic dermatitis. Malzfeldt et al. [4] found that differences in barrier function in the acute inflammatory phase of atopic dermatitis do not influence the efficacy of the glucocorticosteroid preparations since the healing potency of a preparation in which the corticosteroid was suspended was more pronounced in comparison with the drug in a solution type of preparation [2]. In addition, tachyphylaxis must be considered in local corticosteroid therapy, so that a less effective drug would have no effect any longer. It is

Table 4. Weak TCSs (group I)

Generic name	Concentration, %	Brand name	Formulation
Hydrocortisone	0.250	Hydrocortison mild	E
	0.333	Sanatison Mono 1/3%	O
	0.500	Ficortril mite	O
		Ficortril Lotio	Lo
		Hydrocortison Wolff	C, Lo
		Munitren H fettend/fettarm	O
		Velopural	O
	1.000	Ficortril Salbe	O
		Sanatison Mono 1%	O
		Hydrocortison Wolff 1%	C
Hydrocortisone acetate	0.250	Ekzesin	O
	1.000	HC Salbe Mago KG	O
		Sagittacortin	O
		Cordes H	C, O
Prednisolone	0.400	Linola H	E (O/W)
		Linola H fett	E (O/W)
Hydrocortisone	2.000	Ficortril Spray	S
	2.500	Ficortril Salbe 2.5%	O
Fluocortin butylester	0.750	Vaspit	O, C
Triamcinolone acetonide	0.0018	Volonimat Spray	S
Dexamethasone	0.012	Sokaral	Li
	0.030	Anemil mono	O, C
		Cortidexason Crinale	Li
	0.035	Truttozem N Spezial	O
Clocortolone pivalate plus hexanoate each	0.030	Kabanimat	O, C

E = Emulsion; O = ointment; Lo = lotion; C = cream; O/W = oil-in-water; S = spray; Li = liquor.

Table 5. Moderate TCSs (group II)

Generic name	Concentration, %	Brand name	Formulation
Hydrocortisone aceponate	0.100	Retef	O, C
Dexamethasone	0.050	Cortidexason mite	O, C
	0.080	Dexamethason Wolff	C
	0.100	Cortidexason	O
Dexamethasone plus sulfobenzoate each	0.050	Duodexa N	O
Clobetasone butyrate	0.050	Emovate	O, C
Alclometasone dipropionate	0.050	Delonal	O, C
Flumethasone pivalate	0.020	Locacorten	O, C, Lo, Fa
Triamcinolone acetonide	0.0089	Volon A Spray	S
	0.025	Extracort	C
		Volonimat N	O
Fluprednidene acetate	0.050	Decoderm	O
	0.100	Decoderm	C, Lo
		Vobaderm	C, T, P
Fluorandrenolone	0.025	Sermaka 1/2	O, C
Hydrocortisone butyrate	0.100	Alfason	O, C, Li
Hydrocortisone butyrate propionate	0.100	Pandel	O, C
Betamethasone benzoate	0.025	Euvaderm	C
Fluocortolone	0.200	Syracort	O, C
Clocortolone pivalate plus hexanoate each	0.100	Kaban	O, C
Desonide	0.050	Tridesilon	O, C
	0.100	Topifug	C
		Sterax 0.1%	C
Fluorandrenolone	0.050	Sermaka	O, C, Lo, Fo
Betamethasone valerate	0.050	Betnesol-V crinalite	Li
		Betnesol-V mite	O, C
		Celestan-V mite	O, C

Table 5 (continued)

Generic name	Concentra-tion, %	Brand name	Formulation
Triamcinolone acetonide	0.100	Delphicort	O, C
		Kortikoid ratiopharm	O
		Triamcinolon Wolff	C
		Tri-Anemal	O
		Volon A	O, C
Prednicarbate	0.250	Dermatop	O, C
Fluocinolone acetonide	0.010	Jellin Gamma	C
Desoximetasone	0.050	Topisolon mite	O
Halcinonide	0.025	Halcimat	C

O = Ointment; C = cream, Lo = lotion; Fa = foam; S = spray; T = tincture; P = paste, Li = liquor; Fo = foil.

always better to begin with a very potent TCS and withdraw it quickly, instead of instituting a long-lasting therapy with a moderately potent steroid. As soon as the skin improves a TCS of a lower potency should be chosen – the so-called step-down therapy (table 8) [8]; thereafter the amount of TCS has to be reduced by the technique of interval therapy first applying the TCS every other day, then every second and third day, and so on. The treatment during the steroid-free days is done with ointment bases. Thereafter the therapy will be continued with steroid-free ointments, especially with those containing urea.

The weekly application of 25 g of 0.05% topical clobetasol may influence the hypothalamus-pituitary-adrenal axis and the plasma cortisol level, likewise 90 g per week of 0.05% betamethasone dipropionate; however, with up to 105 g per week of 0.25% prednicarbate the plasma cortisol level remains unperturbed [9].

Nonsteroidal Anti-Inflammatory Drugs (NSAIDs) – Bufexamac

The more chronic the inflammatory skin disease the more we need other possible options of treatment. An example for locally applied NSAIDs is bufexa-mac (fig. 1). In vitro, bufexamac inhibits prostaglandin synthesis. The inhibition of inflammation could be demonstrated in several experimental animal models

Table 6. Potent TCSs (group III)

Generic name	Concentration, %	Brand name	Formulation
Betamethasone valerate	0.100	Cordes Beta	O
		Betamethason Wolff	C
		Betnesol-V crinale	Li
		Betnesol-V	O, C, Lo
		Celestan-V crinale	Li
		Celestan-V	O, C
Halomethasone	0.050	Sicorten	O, C
Betamethasone dipropionate	0.050	Diprosone	O, C, Li
		Diprosis	O
Fluocortolone plus hexanoate each	0.250	Ultralan	C, O, S
Fluocinolone acetonide	0.025	Jellin	O, C, Fa, G, Li, Lo
Diflorasone diacetate	0.050	Florone	O, C
Desoximetasone	0.250	Topisolon	O, Lo
Fluocinonide	0.050	Topsym	O, Li
Amcinonide	0.100	Amciderm	O, C
Halcinonide	0.100	Halog	O, Li
Diflucortolone valerate	0.100	Nerisona	O, C

O = Ointment; C = cream; Li = liquor; Lo = lotion; S = spray; Fa = foam; G = gel.

Table 7. Very potent TCSs (group IV)

Generic name	Concentration, %	Brand name	Formulation
Diflucortolone valerate	0.300	Nerisona forte	O
		Temetex forte	O
Clobetasol propionate	0.050	Dermoxinale	Li
		Dermoxin	O, C

O = Ointment; Li = liquor; C = cream.

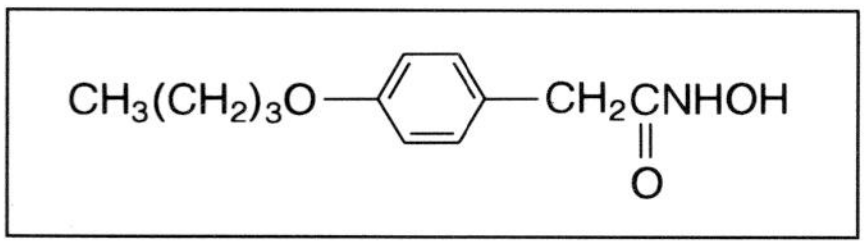

CH$_3$(CH$_2$)$_3$O—⟨benzene⟩—CH$_2$CNHOH
‖
O

Fig. 1. Structure of bufexamac.

Table 8. Step-down and interval therapy

Class IV
      Class III
            Class II
                 Class I
                        ×○×○○×○○×○○×○○○×○○○○○○

×= Treatment with TCS; ○ = treatment with ointment base.

such as UV erythema, carrageenan edema and others. In humans UV erythema was inhibited and the vasoconstriction assay showed an efficacy which corresponded to about 60% of the hydrocortisone effect. In the pyrexal erythema test the efficacy corresponded to that of 0.1–0.5% prednisolone ointment [H.J. Heite, pers. communication, 1977].

The clinical efficacy of bufexamac has been demonstrated in several clinical studies, in practical experience as well as in controlled and randomized double-blind studies [10, 11]. Bufexamac is suitable for mild inflammatory phases or as an additive treatment after corticosteroid therapy. As a side effect an epicutaneous sensitization will occur in 0.1% of cases [12].

Natural Moisturizing Factors (NMFs) – Urea

Yet another possibility for the treatment of eczema is the use of urea, one of the NMFs. In atopic dermatitis a lack of urea can be observed in the skin, in particular in the cornified layer.

Table 9 lists the different properties of urea. Some of these effects depend on the concentration of urea within the respective ointment. A 6% urea ointment is able to split hydrogen bonds, leading to acantholysis of the upper layers of the skin. An 8% urea liquor, applied intracutaneously, produces blisters, and 20% urea ointments will macerate the skin. A keratolytic effect may be seen with 40% urea ointments, which break up the cornified layer by loosening cohesion, separating the cells and dissolving the intercellular matrix [13].

Table 9. Effects of urea

Keratoplastic	Antiproliferative
Keratolytic	Anti-itching
Proteolytic	Promotes the liberation of other substances
Water-binding	Promotes the penetration of other substances
Microbiostatic	Buffering

The antiproliferative effect could be demonstrated by a decrease in ^{3}H-thymidine uptake into epidermal cells; the basal cells were diminished, the time of regeneration of postmitotic cells was prolonged and the cells rested in the metaphase. All these points lead to a thinning of the epidermis of about 20–25% [14].

One of the main effects of urea is the improvement of the waterbinding capacity in the skin. Comparing the effect of a water-in-oil emulsion with a urea-containing one, it could be seen that urea is able to bind much more water in the skin [15]. This effect lasts longer than the application period itself: administered only once, the moisturizing effect lasts for more than 3 h (short-term effect [15]), and administered once a day over a period of 15 days (fig. 2), the effect lasts for more than 10 additional days (long-term effect [16]).

Urea is an ideal agent in the poststeroid treatment phase of inflammatory skin diseases, after having finished the interval therapy. By using urea as monotherapy at a concentration of about 10%, the skin becomes smooth, soft, flexible and nonitching. The penetration of urea into the upper layers of the skin is better when ointments are used instead of creams [13]. A urea cream has an immediate short-lasting effect, compared with a urea ointment showing a delayed but long-lasting effect.

In cases where a mild corticosteroid is needed, hydrocortisone and urea are an ideal combination. Urea is able to promote the liberation of hydrocortisone from its vehicle, as well as its penetration into the skin, because urea weakens the barrier of the horny layer and hydrates it by binding water.

To compare the promotion of hydrocortisone penetration, calculating it on the basis of hydrocortisone alone and giving it a relative penetration factor of 1, the combination of 10% urea plus 1% hydrocortisone results in a factor of 2. The concentration of urea has to be high enough: the higher the urea concentration and the less hydrophilic the vehicle the better the penetration [13].

Clinical studies could prove that the potency of 10% urea plus 1% hydrocortisone is comparable to 0.025% fluocinolone acetonide or 0.1% betamethasone valerate or 0.1% triamcinolone acetonide or 0.05% betamethasone pivalate [17].

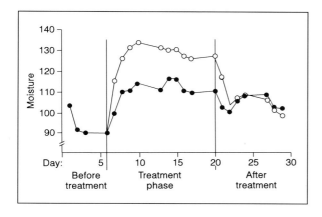

Fig. 2. Moisturizing effect of 10% urea cream (○). ● = Placebo.

High-Dose Ultraviolet A-1 Irradiation

An alternative treatment for atopic dermatitis is the use of UV irradiation. It is well known that the combination of UVB with UVA irradiation is more effective than UVB alone [18]. So it may be supposed that UVA alone is of benefit in the treatment of this disease, but, because of the relatively low dose of UVA, several weeks of treatment are required to observe an improvement in atopic dermatitis. In order to see the benefit more quickly, much higher doses of UVA are needed, which had to be free of UVB.

As demonstrated in figure 3, high-dose UVA-1 irradiation leads to a significant decrease in the severity score (36.4 ± 1.7 before vs. 8.9 ± 1.1 after therapy; p < 0.001). A comparable result is demonstrated in figure 4 [19], where the overall clinical score shows a rapid improvement in atopic dermatitis (53.0 ± 1.9 before vs. 14.0 ± 3.2 after therapy; p < 0.001). Six high-dose UVA-1 exposures were sufficient to reduce the severity score by about 50%, suggesting a fast-acting therapeutic mechanism. No serious side effects were observed in either group; only slight erythema caused by overexposure was noticed with UVA/UVB therapy.

What are the potential mechanisms for the effectiveness of high-dose UVA-1 therapy? This question cannot be separated from the questions regarding the relevant pathomechanisms of atopic dermatitis. At the beginning of the 1980s the immunomodulating effects of UVB irradiation were discovered [20]. The antigen-presenting cells of the epidermis, the Langerhans cells, are an important target of UVB irradiation. UVB leads to a reduction of Langerhans cell markers and partially inhibits the function of human antigen-presenting cells [21, 22]. Thus, it is an interesting point that patients with atopic dermatitis who underwent therapy with UVB showed a reduction of their normally increased Langerhans cells in the epidermis. Recent investigations could demonstrate that the intercellular adhe-

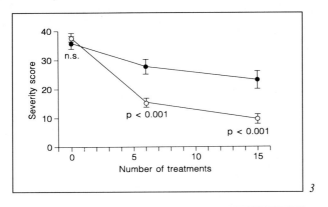

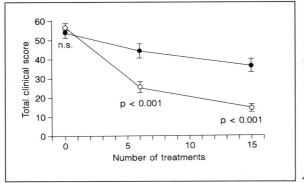

Fig. 3. Changes in severity score during treatment with high-dose UVA-1 (○) and UVA/UVB (●) therapy.

Fig. 4. Changes in total clinical score during treatment with high-dose UVA-1 (○) and UVA/UVB (●) therapy.

sion molecule 1 (ICAM-1) is an important target for UVB-induced immunosuppression [21], and that UVB inhibits significantly the cytokine-induced ICAM-1 expression in human keratinocytes. Langerhans cells, keratinocytes and T lymphocytes are target cells for PUVA therapy. Although there are no exact data about the mode of action of high-dose UVA-1 therapy, it may be speculated that these target cells may be of importance in this kind of therapy, too, as seen by the treatment with UVB and PUVA. It seems as if there were important differences, considering the significantly better effects and the rapid onset of benefits.

Besides all this, the elevated serum levels of eosinophilic cationic protein decrease significantly under therapy with high-dose UVA-1. Serum eosinophilic cationic protein may be a marker for the severity of atopic dermatitis. The decrease may not reflect a direct effect of high-dose UVA-1 on eosinophil function but may only indicate that the activity of atopic dermatitis decreases under this therapy [19].

References

1 Cornell RC, Maibach HI: Clinical indications: Real and assumed; in Maibach HI, Surber Ch (eds): Topical corticosteroids. Basel, Karger, 1992, pp 154–162.
2 Goerz G, Lehmann P: Topical treatment with corticosteroids; in Ruzicka T, Ring J, Przybilla B (eds): Handbook of Atopic Eczema. Berlin, Springer, 1991, pp 375–390.
3 Surber Ch, Maibach HI: The Future; in Maibach HI, Surber Ch (eds): Topical Corticosteroids. Basel, Karger, 1992, pp 227–234.
4 Malzfeldt E, Lehmann P, Goerz G, Lippold PC: Drug solubility in vehicle and efficacy of ointments. Arch Dermatol Res 1989;281:193–197.
5 Stoughton RB: Vasoconstrictor assay – Specific applications; in Maibach HI, Surber Ch (eds): Topical Corticosteroids. Basel, Karger, 1992, pp 42–53.
6 Niedner R: Extern anzuwendende Glukokortikosteroide. Teil 1: Anwendungsregeln – Klassifikation. Fortschr Med 1992;110:327–329.
7 Schalla W: Lokaltherapie mit Kortikoiden. Z Hautkr 1985;60:609–618.
8 Pflugshaupt C: Diskontinuierliche topische Corticoidtherapie. Z Haut Geschlechtskr 1983;148:1229–1238.
9 Ernst TM: Reaktion der körpereigenen Cortisolproduktion bei Patienten mit ausgedehnter Psoriasis oder ausgedehnter atopischer Dermatitis nach externer Applikation einer Fettsalbe von Prednicarbat (0.25%). Z Hautkr 1989;64(suppl 1):28–34.
10 Kohnosu M: Results of clinical application of bufexamac cream. Clin Rep (Jap) 1972;6:258–264.
11 Schittko I: Parfenac Salbe als alternative Therapie zu Kortikoiden bei Hauterkrankungen im Säuglingsalter. Therapiewoche 1979;29:5963–5966.
12 Klaschka K: Stellenwert eines nicht-steroidalen Externums: Darstellung experimenteller und klinischer Ergebnisse. Dtsch Dermatol 1987;35:52–57.
13 Wohlrab W: Therapie der «trockenen Haut» mit harnstoffhaltigen Externa. Z Hautkr 1988;63(suppl 3):20–23.
14 Wohlrab W: Bedeutung von Harnstoff in der externen Therapie. Hautarzt 1988;40(suppl IX):35–41.
15 Taube KM: Feuchthalteeffekt und Verträglichkeit von harnstoffhaltigen Externa bei Neurodermitikern. Hautarzt 1992;43(suppl XI):30–32.
16 Puschmann M, Gogoll K: Verbesserung der Hautfeuchte und des Hautreliefs unter Harnstofftherapie. Hautarzt 1989;40(suppl IX):67–70.
17 Ernst TM: Zur Wirkungssteigerung des Hydrocortisons unter Harnstoffzusatz. Z Hautkr 1980;55:806–812.
18 Jekler J, Larkö O: Combined UV-A-UV-B versus UV-B phototherapy for atopic dermatitis: A paired-comparison study. J Am Acad Dermatol 1990;22:49–53.
19 Krutmann J, Czech W, Diepgen T, Niedner R, Kapp A, Schöpf E: High-dose UVA1 therapy in the treatment of patients with atopic dermatitis. J Am Acad Dermatol 1992;26:225–230.
20 Stingl G: Ultraviolettlicht und epidermale Immunphänomene. Hautarzt 1984;35:121–125.
21 Krutmann J, Kammer GM, Toosie Z, Waller R, Ellner JJ, Elmets CA: UVB irradiation and human monocyte accessory function: Differential effects on premitotic events in T-cell activation. J Invest Dermatol 1990;94:204–209.
22 Simon JC, Cruz PD, Bergstresser PR, Tigelaar RE: Low-dose UVB-irradiated Langerhans cells (LC) preferentially activate CD4+ T cells of the TH$_2$ subset. J Immunol 1990;145:2087–2091.

Prof. Dr. med. R. Niedner, Universitäts-Hautklinik, Hauptstrasse 7,
D–79104 Freiburg i.Br. (FRG)

Korting HC, Maibach HI (eds): Topical Glucocorticoids with Increased Benefit/Risk Ratio.
Curr Probl Dermatol. Basel, Karger, 1993, vol 21, pp 170–179

....

Contact Allergy to Topical Glucocorticoids

Peter Elsner

Department of Dermatology, University of Zurich, Switzerland

Glucocorticoids are important therapeutic substances used for the suppression of both antibody- and cell-mediated immunologic reactions. They may be used systemically and topically on mucous membranes and the skin. Although glucocorticoids serve as inhibitors of allergic reactions, they may be allergens themselves. Since their introduction into clinical use a wide range of allergic reactions to glucocorticoids have been described (table 1). These reactions may be of type I (IgE-mediated) or of type IV (cell-mediated) according to Gell and Coombs.

Only a few years after the introduction of topical corticosteroids into dermatotherapy [1] the first case of delayed-type contact allergy to hydrocortisone was reported by Burckhardt in 1959 [2]. Since then, nearly 200 cases of contact dermatitis from corticosteroids have been reported. Systematic screening studies, however, have only been performed in recent years.

Mechanisms of Corticosteroid Allergy

Very little is known about the mechanisms by which corticosteroid derivates may become allergens. As for the relationship between chemical structure and allergenicity, Rivara et al. [3] speculated that the C_{17} substituent, an acetate group in position 21 and the dienone system of ring A may be the electrophilic sites where skin nucleophilic proteins may attack and thus transform haptens to full antigens. Wilkinson and English [4] tested 11 patients positive on patch testing to tixocortol pivalate with a series of hydrocortisone analogues intradermally. While substitution of C_{21} had no effect on the frequency of positive reactions to hydrocortisone, changes in the carbon rings altered cross-reactivity considerably.

Table 1. Allergic reactions to glucocorticosteroids

Type of allergy (according to Gell and Coombs)	Clinical symptoms
Type I (humoral, IgE-mediated)	urticaria, angioedema rhinitis laryngitis asthma anaphylactic shock
Type IV (cellular)	contact dermatitis drug exanthema

Regarding immunologic mechanisms in corticosteroid allergy, Lauerma et al. [5] recently showed that skin Langerhans cells, but not blood macrophages, are capable of presenting corticosteroids to T lymphocytes from patients with corticosteroid hypersensitivity, resulting in T cell proliferation.

Methodological Problems in Patch Testing Corticosteroids

Before a corticosteroid allergy is considered when a patient does not seem to tolerate a topical corticosteroid, a sensitization to a noncorticoid component in the product should be considered and excluded. Fisher [6] mentions ethylenediamine hydrochloride, parabens, benzyl alcohol, isopropyl palmitate, stearyl alcohol, propylene glycol and polysorbate 60 as possible allergens that may be present in commercial corticosteroid preparations. When commercial topical corticosteroids are used for patch testing and positive reactions are encountered, the components of the product should be obtained from the manufacturer and tested separately.

Regarding the patch test conditions of corticosteroids, there has been a considerable and still ongoing debate in the literature. Obviously, the anti-inflammatory effect of glucocorticosteroids may suppress allergic contact dermatitis and it may thus hide an allergic patch test reaction. It has, therefore, been proposed to test corticosteroids in higher concentrations than used for commercial preparations. Furthermore, the vehicle of commercial creams and ointments is generally optimized to high percutaneous penetration of the substance. This is not the case for standard patch test vehicles. While the commercial preparations are usually preserved to prevent significant degradation of the corticosteroid during the guaranteed usage period, corticosteroid substances may show considerable decay both in petrolatum and in ethanol. Therefore, custom-made corticosteroid patch test solutions should be kept in the refrigerator and should be renewed frequently.

In our own experience, there are no relevant differences in the severity of reactions to commercial preparations and to the pure corticosteroids tested in concentrations up to 100 times higher than the commercial preparations [7]. Since at the moment no patch test preparations for frequently used topical corticosteroids are commercially available, we recommend testing as is with the product the patient has used. If a positive reaction is observed, we test with the pure substance obtained from the manufacturer.

In reading patch tests with corticosteroids, one encounters not infrequently 'irritant' reactions, i.e. erythema and edema of the test area that do rapidly decrease with time. On repeated patch tests, these reactions are often not reproducible. In addition to irritation, these reactions may have a pharmacologic background. Topical corticosteroids cause vasoconstriction of skin blood vessels that may be followed by vasodilation clinically visible as erythema when the corticoid effect ceases. It is important not to read these phenomena as positive allergic patch test reactions which will develop later (72 or 96 h, sometimes even 144 h) and consist of erythema, papules and possibly vesicles.

The Choice of Screening Substances for Corticosteroid Allergy

In order to screen for corticosteroid allergy on a routine basis, it would be useful to have a set of screening substances. In 1986, Dooms-Gossens et al. [8] reported the case of a patient sensitive to pure hydrocortisone who also reacted to tixocortol pivalate. This was noteworthy since tixocortol pivalate was not on the Belgian market at that time and an independent sensitization could be thus excluded. Tixocortol pivalate has since been shown to be a strong sensitizer in the guinea pig maximization assay [9] and to sensitize humans after only a few days of mucosal application [10]. The substance was therefore proposed as a marker for sensitization to certain other corticosteroids. Tixocortol pivalate has been used in several studies as a screening substance and it was superior to hydrocortisone in detecting corticosteroid allergy [8, 11–13]. Unfortunately, tixocortol pivalate is not commercially available as a pure substance, but only as a nasal spray (Pivalone®). Lauerma [13] recently proposed the combination of 0.1% tixocortol pivalate as a 1/10 mixture of Pivalone nasal spray in ethanol with 1.0% hydrocortisone 17-butyrate in ethanol for screening purposes.

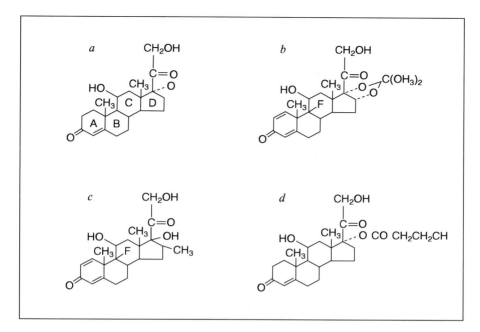

Fig. 1. Allergologic corticosteroid classes as proposed by Coopman and Dooms-Gossens [14] and Coopman et al. [15]. *a* Class A. Hydrocortisone type: no substitution on D or C-17 chain; including C_{17}- and/or C_{21}-acetate ester and tixocortol pivalate. *b* Class B. Triamcinolone type: C_{16}, C_{17}-*cis*,-diol or -ketal chain. *c* Class C. Betamethasone type: C_{16}-alkyl substitution. *d* Class D. Hydrocortisone 17-butyrate type: long-chain ester at C-17 and/or C-21 position.

Cross-Reactions between Topical Corticosteroids

Recently, Coopman and Dooms-Gossens [15] delineated 4 classes (A–D) of chemically related corticosteroids (fig. 1a–d). Based on a literature review and their own patch test data, they concluded that positive patch tests to corticosteroids occur 6–7 times more frequently within these classes than between corticosteroids from different classes. In our own experience, the concept of allergologic corticosteroid classes is of limited values in predicting sensitizations to other molecules in patients sensitized to one corticosteroid [7]. This may be due to the fact that our allergologic high-risk patients are frequently independently cosensitized to other corticosteroids.

In the Department of Dermatology, University of Würzburg, FRG, we patch tested patients who noticed worsening of their dermatosis after using topical glucocorticoid preparations [7]. Between 1987 and 1989, 10 cases of contact derma-

Table 2. Patch-test-proven cases of topical corticosteroid sensitization in the Department of Dermatology, University of Würzburg, 1987–1989

Patient No.	Age years	Sex	Underlying skin disease	Corticosteroid responsible for contact dermatitis
1	68	f	leg ulcers	amcinonide
2	36	f	psoriasis	amcinonide
3	48	m	chronic dermatitis	hydrocortisone butyrate
4	41	f	leg ulcer	clobetasol 17-propionate
5	62	m	stasis dermatitis	clobetasol 17-propionate
6	22	m	chronic dermatitis	betamethasone valerate
7	77	f	leg ulcers	prednicarbate
8	57	m	chronic dermatitis	betamethasone valerate
9	60	m	chronic dermatitis	fluocortolone
10	45	f	chronic dermatitis	fluocortolone

titis due to topical glucocorticoids were observed (table 2). The corticosteroid allergens were amcinonide (2 patients), hydrocortisone butyrate, clobetasol propionate (2), betamethasone valerate (2), prednicarbate and fluocortolone (2). 9 of the patients were patch tested with a corticosteroid series that included compounds of all 4 corticosteroid classes according to Coopman et al. [15]. In all of the 9 patients, reactions to further corticosteroids were observed (table 3). However, these possible cross-reactions were not restricted to substances within the corticosteroid class of the primary allergen, but they were also observed to corticoids in different classes.

Independent sensitizations to the latter substances could not be ruled out, since the patients may have used them without recalling. Nevertheless, this patient series demonstrates that the concept of allergologic corticosteroid classes may be of academic interest, but it is of doubtful value in clinical practice as any corticosteroid must be considered a potential allergen in this high-risk population.

Frequency of Type IV Sensitizations to Corticosteroids

Most of the data on corticosteroid sensitizations available in the literature are case reports. Prospective studies in large patient populations are rare. Even the information on larger populations that is available is probably influenced by the heterogeneity of patient populations tested in different centers. Although this

Table 3. Patch test reactions to further corticosteroid classes A–D according to Coopman et al. [15] in the patients of table 2

Patient No.	Patch test reactions to corticosteroid class			
	A	B	C	D
1[a]		+		
2		+(+)		
3		(+)		+
4	(+)			+
5		(+)	(+)	+
6		(+)		+
7		(+)		+(+)
8		(+)	(+)	+(+)
9			+(+)	
10			+(+)	

+ = Reaction to corticosteroid responsible for contact dermatitis in the patient; (+) = reaction to further corticosteroids in the patch test series.
[a] Patient No. 1 was only tested with his own corticosteroid, but not with further steroids in the patch test series.

is true for most patch test data, it marks a failure to collect the information that is necessary to characterize test populations and to make the results of prevalence studies comparable with other investigations. Differences in test populations together with variations in test protocols and reading procedures may thus account to a great part for the divergence in the published prevalence data.

Alani and Alani [16] included corticosteroids when patch testing 1,843 patients with contact dermatitis. They saw 21 positive reactions to hydrocortisone (1.1%), 3 to triamcinolone, 2 to betamethasone and 10 to pure hydrocortisone.

In a study of 1,906 patients suspected of corticosteroid allergy tested between 1984 and 1986, Dooms-Gossens [17] found 6 patients (0.3%) with contact sensitivity to certain corticosteroids. In 471 routine patch test patients tested in 1987, she identified 8 cases of tixocortol pivalate allergy (1.7%).

In 1989, the European Environmental and Contact Dermatitis Research Group performed a multicenter screening study with tixocortol pivalate [11]. 4,319 consecutive patients were tested with 1% tixocortol pivalate in petrolatum.

Table 4. Corticosteroid screening series of the SCDRG multicenter study

Tixocortol pivalate	1% petrolatum
Hydrocortisone acetate	1.5% ethanol
Budesonide	1% petrolatum
Hydrocortisone butyrate	1% ethanol

Table 5. Extended corticosteroid screening series of the SCDRG multicenter study

Amcinonide	1% petrolatum
Betamethasone valerate	5% petrolatum
Betamethasone dipropionate	5% petrolatum
Clobetasol propionate	0.5% petrolatum
Desoximethasone	1% petrolatum
Diflucortolone valerate	1% petrolatum
Flumethasone pivalate	1% petrolatum
Flucinonide	1% petrolatum
Halcinonide	1% petrolatum
Halomethasone	1% petrolatum
Prednisolone	5% petrolatum
Triamcinolone acetate	1% petrolatum

83 (1.9%) reacted with a variation in frequency from 0.2% (Barcelona) to 3.4% (Belfast, Oulu). 42 of these 83 tixocortol-pivalate-positive patients were tested with 0.5 and 0.1% dilutions of the substance. 39 of them reacted positively which is in favor of an allergic reaction.

Lauerma [13] reported about a prospective study in 727 patch test clinic patients tested with hydrocortisone, tixocortol pivalate and hydrocortisone 17-butyrate. 28 patients (3.9%) reacted to tixocortol pivalate, 10 (1.4%) to hydrocortisone 17-butyrate and 2 (0.4%) to hydrocortisone.

Wilkinson et al. [18] tested intradermally for hydrocortisone allergy and found a sensitization rate of 4.8%. Goldermann et al. [19] patch tested 60 patients with suspected allergic contact dermatitis with a corticoid series proposed by the German Contact Allergy Group. Seven patients (12%) showed positive reactions to corticosteroid preparations. In 4 cases, these were due to noncorticoid compounds in the ointments, especially to parabens. Three patients (5%) remained with contact allergy to corticosteroids.

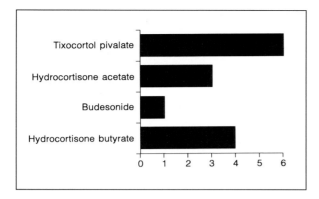

Fig. 2. Patch test reactions to corticoid screening allergens (Patch Test Laboratory of the Department of Dermatology, University of Zurich, n = 787).

In an ongoing multicenter study of the Swiss Contact Dermatitis Research Group (SCDRG; study coordinator: A. Bircher, Basel), we are screening all patients tested with the standard series for corticosteroid allergy. The substances of the screening series are shown in table 4. When positive patch test reactions are observed, the patients are retested with the screening series and tested with an extended corticosteroid series (table 5) and possibly with their own products. Positive reactions are finally confirmed with a repeated open application test to establish relevance. In the Department of Dermatology, University of Zurich, 787 patients were screened during a 6-month period between November 1991 and April 1992. Only 6 patients (0.76%) remained positive in the confirmation test (fig. 2). 1 patient (0.13%) showed positive reactions in the extended series. The positive reactions were considered relevant in 2 patients (0.26% of all tested or one third of the test-positives).

Patient Populations at Risk for Corticosteroid Sensitizations

Although risk populations have not been exactly defined according to epidemiologic criteria, it is safe to state that the patients at risk of developing corticosteroid contact allergy are those suffering from chronic dermatitis requiring topical therapy over an extended period, especially those with stasis dermatitis and leg ulcers and patients with chronic contact dermatitis. These patients are often allergic to further substances such as cream bases, emulsifiers and further topical preparations.

Sensitizing Potential of Single Corticosteroids

As summarized above, tixocortol pivalate seems to be a potent sensitizer based on animal and human data. For other corticosteroids, this amount of information is not available. While a literature search reveals case reports on sensitizations to almost any corticosteroid molecule, this information is epidemiologically useless since no data on the modes and frequency of application in a defined population are available which would be essential to estimate the sensitization capacity of specific substances. These reservations hold also true for a study based on the spontaneous reporting system of the German Medical Association [20]. Since spontaneous reporting may be heavily influenced by nonmedical factors such as the introduction of new products into the market associated with a higher physician awareness of side effects, it remains uncertain if the newer corticoids amcinonide and prednicarbate are more frequent causes of contact dermatitis than other corticosteroids as reported in this study. On the other hand, there are no published data that would indicate a decreased sensitization potential of the newer corticosteroids with increased benefit/risk ratio.

Conclusion

There are considerable discrepancies in the reported prevalence of type IV allergies to corticosteroids. These discrepancies may be explained by different usage patterns, as well as by differences in test populations, in the corticoid substances used for testing, in test methods, in the reading of reactions and variations in confirmation procedures. In our experience, relevant sensitizations to glucocorticoids are rare in nonselected patch test populations, whereas patients with chronic dermatitis and leg ulcers seem to be at increased risk for corticosteroid allergy.

A careful review of the literature reveals that practically any glucocorticosteroid may be a type IV allergen. There is agreement that certain substances such as tixocortol pivalate are relatively potent allergens that may be used for screening purposes. Allergic reactions have also been observed to the so-called fourth generation corticosteroids such as prednicarbate. Current data are inadequate to decide whether these newer compounds are different from older ones regarding their sensitization potential.

Acknowledgment

The author would like to acknowledge the skilful technical assistance of Ms. Petra Halm, Patch Test Laboratory of the Department of Dermatology, University of Zurich.

References

1 Sulzberger MB, Witten VH: The effect of topically applied compound F in selected dermatoses. J Invest Dermatol 1952;18:101–102.
2 Burckhardt W: Kontaktekzem durch Hydrocortison. Hautarzt 1959;10:42–43.
3 Rivara G, Tomb RR, Foussereau J: Allergic contact dermatitis from topical corticosteroids. Contact Dermatitis 1989;21:83–91.
4 Wilkinson SM, English JSC: Hydrocortisone sensitivity: An investigation into the nature of the allergen. Contact Dermatitis 1991;25:178–181.
5 Lauerma AI, Rasanen L, Reunala T, Reitamo S: Langerhans cells but not monocytes are capable of antigen presentation in vitro in corticosteroid contact hypersensitivity. Br J Dermatol 1990;123: 699–705.
6 Fisher AA: Contact Dermatitis. Philadelphia, Lea & Febiger, 1986.
7 Dunkel FG, Elsner P, Burg G: Contact allergies to topical corticosteroids: 10 cases of contact dermatitis. Contact Dermatitis 1991;25:97–103.
8 Dooms-Gossens A, Verscheave H, Degreef H, van Beerendonks J: Contact allergy to hydrocortisone and tixocortol pivalate: Problems in the detection of corticosteroid sensitivity. Contact Dermatitis 1986;14:94–102.
9 Hausen BM, Foussereau J: The sensitizing capacity of tixocortol pivalate. Contact Dermatitis 1988; 18:63–64.
10 Bircher AJ: Short induction phase of contact allergy to tixocortol pivalate in a nasal spray. Contact Dermatitis 1990;22:237–238.
11 Dooms-Gossens A, Andersen KE, Burrows D, et al: A survey of the results of patch tests with tixocortol pivalate. Contact Dermatitis 1989;20:158.
12 Wilkinson SM, English JSC: Hydrocortisone sensitivity: A prospective study of the value of tixocortol pivalate and hydrocortisone acetate as patch test markers. Contact Dermatitis 1991;25:132–133.
13 Lauerma AI: Screening for corticosteroid contact sensitivity: Comparison of tixocortol pivalate, hydrocortisone-17-butyrate and hydrocortisone. Contact Dermatitis 1991;24:123–130.
14 Coopman S, Dooms-Gossens A: Cross-reactions in topical corticosteroid contact dermatitis. Contact Dermatitis 1988;19:145–146.
15 Coopman S, Degreef H, Dooms GA: Identification of cross-reaction patterns in allergic contact dermatitis from topical corticosteroids. Br J Dermatol 1989;121:27–34.
16 Alani MD, Alani SD: Allergic contact dermatitis to corticosteroids. Ann Allergy 1972;30:181.
17 Dooms-Gossens A: Identification of undetected corticosteroid allergy. Contact Dermatitis 1988;18: 124–125.
18 Wilkinson SM, Cartwright PH, English JSC: Hydrocortisone: An important cutaneous allergen. Lancet 1991;337:761–762.
19 Goldermann R, Teilkemeier P, Lehmann P, Goerz G: Typ-IV-Sensibilisierung gegen Kortikoide. Z Hautkr 1992;67:430–435.
20 Hopf G, Mathias B: Glukokortikoid-Externa und Kontaktdermatitis. Münch Med Wochenschr 1989;131:595–599.

Priv.-Doz. Dr. P. Elsner, Department of Dermatology, University of Zurich, Gloriastrasse 31, CH–8091 Zürich (Switzerland)

Korting HC, Maibach HI (eds): Topical Glucocorticoids with Increased Benefit/Risk Ratio.
Curr Probl Dermatol. Basel, Karger, 1993, vol 21, pp 180–185

Adverse Drug Reactions to Various Topical Glucocorticosteroids: Quantitative Aspects

Th. Höhler, K. Wörz, V. Himmler

Clinical Research Department, Cassella-Riedel Pharma GmbH,
Frankfurt/Main, FRG

Adequate consideration of the quantitative aspects of adverse drug reactions (ADRs) due to topical glucocorticosteroids (GCS) requires a multidisciplinary approach and necessitates support from biometrics and drug safety departments. The subject is further complicated by the fact that there is no officially accepted methodology for the assessment of risk-benefit ratio [1]. A definition and discussion of the methodology and terminology involved is beyond the scope of this paper which places emphasis on a review of the information about quantitative aspects of ADRs due to topical use of GCS available. A book publication is expected in the near future that should deal with methods of risk-benefit analysis in detail [1].

This presentation will not discuss the qualitative aspects of GCS ADRs, a subject which has been dealt with by a number of papers [e.g., 2–4]. In addition to this we have to note that very severe ADRs to topical GCS have been reported occasionally in the literature. Dhein [5], for example, describes the dramatic development of full-blown striae on the trunk of a patient using 100 g ointment of a very potent fluorinated GCS preparation per week over a period of 12 months. This young man also developed Cushing's syndrome. Such extreme cases of abuse are thankfully very rare.

On reviewing the available literature, we came across an editorial in the *Lancet* from 1977 entitled 'The hazardous jungle of topical steroid' [6] and were interested to see whether a more detailed analysis would substantiate this image.

In theory, the definition of risk potential involves establishing which events are ADRs and how frequently they occur [7]. In reality, the situation is much more complicated. It may be extremely difficult for the individual doctor to assess the causal relationship of an event in a given patient to that patient's medication.

In addition, it is also difficult to obtain exact/valid data on the frequency of use of a medication. With respect to topical GCS, the quality of ADRs are fairly well defined. There is a list of 20 (or more) ADRs [cf. references in 1–3], which are attributed to topical GCS. But how frequently do these occur?

There are several methods for obtaining data on adverse drug reactions [8]. The two most frequently used methods are the spontaneous adverse drug reaction recording systems and phase V studies or post-marketing surveillance as favored by pharmaceutical companies [9]. The latter is important in establishing, during say the first 1 million treatment cycles with a new drug, how frequently ADRs might occur, which could cause withdrawal of the drug from the market [10].

The problems associated with spontaneous reporting systems are illustrated by the previous paper with reference to allergies reported to the German Drug Commission. The inherent difficulties in spontaneous reporting are also highlighted in a publication by Avron [11]. The number of ADRs reported might depend on how recently the drug was introduced, how widely it is used, its labelling and the sort of 'press' it obtains in the literature. The effects of drug labelling on ADR reporting are illustrated by an example given by Urquhart [10]. Indometacin was introduced as an osmotic slow-release form with the claim that it is very safe in patients who had a history of gastrointestinal problems taking nonsteroidal anti-inflammatory drugs. As a result, the drug was administered to problem patients and doctors were more aware of unwanted gastrointestinal effects. The drug was subsequently accused of producing gastrointestinal ulcers and withdrawn from the market due to the number of reports of severe side effects. However, the number of such ADRs on plain indometacin is still not clear! This is an example of drug channelling through labelling and illustrates how spontaneous ADE reporting can be influenced. On a more positive note, Hoigné and Hottinger [8] as well as Scott et al. [12] were able to demonstrate that the establishment of a spontaneous reporting system, providing support for the doctors, increases the 'normally' low to very low reporting frequency.

Although special studies are a good source of ADR data, the fact that they represent selected populations must be borne in mind otherwise they can be misleading with respect to frequency. This is demonstrated e.g. by data from a special study reported by Günther [13]. The selected population was composed of 111 individuals (59 m, 52 f) from 2 to 15 years of age hospitalized in Germany in 1976, who had problems with long-term use of topical and/or systemic GCS. 59/60 patients using only topical GCS had severe ADRs including Cushing's syndrome and growth retardation (5% of patients each).

In other publications such as that by Akers [14] reporting controlled clinical trials with topical GCS, the overall incidence of ADRs is relatively low (4.4% of 5,698 treatment exposures). The majority of these were unspecific, i.e. not specific for GCS-induced adverse reactions and this seems to be fairly representative

Table 1. Skin damage caused by prolonged use of topical GCS – a statistical analysis (from Hornstein et al. [15]; also see references cited in Akers [14]): one year screening (06/73–05/74) of 7,978 newly seen patients (ADRs excluded: pathomorphosis; secondary infections) – results show ADRs found in 75 patients (49 f, 26 m)

Teleangiectasias – rubeosis	46%	Steroid acne	6%
Epidermal atrophies	16%	Purpura	3%
Hypertrichosis	9%	Atrophies, cut./subcut.	3%
Striae	8%	Others	2%
Milia	7%		

of well controlled clinical studies. The GCS-specific side effects occurred at a frequency of less than 1:1,000. In general, the ADRs in the series of studies reviewed by Akers were mild, transient and rare.

As far as we are aware, the only publication on the epidemiology of topical GCS-induced ADRs allowing the construction of a quantitative ADR profile is the one by Hornstein et al. [15]. A review of a population of approximately 8,000 patients attending the Erlangen Department of Dermatology in Germany from June 1973 to May 1974 is given. The results obtained in this study (table 1) will be considered as a standard against which to measure the profiles of individual GCS substances. GCS-associated ADRs were observed in 75 individuals (approx. 1%) from this relatively large population and most of the patients with ADRs had a long history of topical GCS use. As can be seen from table 1, the most frequent ADRs were teleangiectasias and rubeosis and there were no severe systemic ADRs in this population. 46% of the 75 patients presented with side effects relating to the atrophy-inducing potential of GCS, although the incidence would probably be higher if the relatively mild atrophies of the epidermis were included.

These data can be put into perspective by comparing them with the incidence of skin side effects of very well-known drugs [16]. Aminopenicillins, allopurinol, and nonsteroidal anti-inflammatory drugs, all can induce an exanthema after exposure. Aminopenicillins induce a higher rate of topical effects (approx. 7.7%), allopurinol, a well-known treatment for gout, causes an almost similar frequency (approx. 1.1%), although the absolute numbers are low, while analgesics and non-steroidal anti-inflammatory drugs cause a little less (approx. 0.4%) than GCS.

Table 2 compares the ADR profiles of prednicarbate observed in controlled and open clinical trials and reported spontaneously with spontaneous reports of ADRs on desoxymethasone. The number of treatment cycles which were responsible for the spontaneous reports of ADRs due to prednicarbate has been estimated at 4 million, but due to the uncertainties involved, the number probably lies somewhere between 3 and 5 million. The first thing to note is that the overall

Table 2. ADRs from clinical trials and as spontaneous reports: topical GCS prednicarbate and desoxymethasone – absolute numbers and relative frequencies of GCS-specific events

	Clinical trials	Spontaneous reports	
	prednicarbate 0.25% n/N: 20/16.092 (0.12%)	prednicarbate 0.25% n/N: 39/approx. 4 million (approx. 0.2‰)[1]	desoxy- methasone 0.25% n = 48
Folliculitis	8	4	–
Skin atrophy	4	4	6
Discoloration	3	–	11
Acne	2	10	7
Hirsutism (local)	1	2	–
Purpura	1	–	2
Perioral dermatitis	1	19	4
Striae	–	–	10
Cushing	–	–	5
Weight gain	–	–	2
Gynecomastia	–	–	1

[1] Calculated under the assumption that only 5% of ADRs are reported spontaneously.

frequency of ADRs in clinical trials is down about one order of magnitude from that reported in 1975 by Hornstein et al. [15]. Due to the low numbers involved it is not possible to determine whether the frequencies of the single signs and symptoms of ADRs are actually different. Nevertheless, the atrophy-related ADRs are only one third as compared to the standard. However, the profile of spontaneously reported ADRs due to desoxymethasone is different to that due to prednicarbate, the most obvious difference being the absence of striae and Cushing's syndrome with prednicarbate. One marked difference between the spontaneous reports of ADRs due to prednicarbate and those observed in clinical trials is the number of cases of perioral dermatitis. This ADR was reported in 19 of the 39 patients (49%) who were subject of spontaneous reports. This might be a drug-channelling effect, but the very low numbers involved cannot allow more than the suspicion of a trend. Since perioral dermatitis is no indication for GCS treatment, the ADR nature of these events is unclear and might be regarded as misuse.

Urquhart [10] proposed the rule of 200 for the calculation of how often ADRs occur on a statistical base. This is an empirical rule, which simply states that the number of patients without ADRs divided by 200 gives the probability of ADRs with 95% confidence limits. Bearing in mind all of the difficulties of spontaneous reporting systems, the frequency registered for prednicarbate is still one order of magnitude beyond the calculated figure (0.5%).

A review of the literature was performed in an attempt to determine whether there had been a change in the frequency of ADRs on topical GCS from the 1970s to the 1980s. The specific question which we wanted to address was: Is the lower frequency of prednicarbate ADRs related to the properties of the drug or to changes in the behavior of the physicians/patients in reporting these reactions?

From Germany we can gain access to 2,100 of the 6,414 commercial data bases worldwide through 64 hosts. For our purposes DataStar appeared suitable, because some 60% of the total data volume in this host is concerned with medical literature. In the 7 million documents available on Medline for the period 1966–1992, there are 400,000 (5.7%) on ADRs. GCS are cited 20,373 times and in 1,235 of these there are citations of GCS and ADRs (6.1%). Topical GCS are cited 846 times and 25% of these (213 citations) concerned ADRs. When these 213 papers were analyzed for key word frequencies, it was not possible to obtain a good quantitative profile of ADRs and the numbers were too low to enable a comparison of the ADR frequencies in the 1970s, 80s or 90s. Thus, this method was unable to generate the data necessary for an adequate comparison. The main conclusion that we can draw from this exercise is that this method is probably less sensitive than the spontaneous reporting system, which, in extreme cases, is believed to collect data on about 5% of the severe drug reactions only which actually occur. Since the ADRs of topical GCS are mostly moderate and infrequent, the spontaneous system might not give better results for this class of drugs.

In conclusion, it can be stated that, based on the available literature and on our own first-hand experience, it is clear that there are very severe cases of ADRs. However, these are very rare and a 'normal' frequency can be estimated as between 0.1 and 1% of the total number of treatment cycles.

In the case of the spontaneous ADR reports for prednicarbate, based on 100% estimation (39 cases = 5%, see table 2) a rate of 0.2‰ was established in approximately 4 million treatment cycles.

References

1   Victor N, Schäfer H, Nowak H: Arzneimittelforschung nach der Zulassung: Bestandsaufnahme und Perspektiven; in Überla K, Rienhoff O, Victor V (eds): Medizinische Informatik und Statistik, vol 73. Berlin, Springer, in press.
2   Schöpf E: Side effects from topical corticosteroid therapy. Ann Clin Res 1975;7:353–367.
3   Kligman AM: Adverse effects of topical corticosteroids; in Christophers E, Schöpf E, Kligman AM, Stoughton RB (eds): Topical Corticosteroid Therapy – A Novel Approach to Safer Drugs. New York, Raven Press, 1988, pp 181–187.
4   Marks R: Adverse side effects from the use of topical corticosteroids; in Maibach H, Surber Ch (eds): Topical Corticosteroids. Basel, Karger, 1992, pp 170–183.

5   Dhein S: Cushing's syndrome after topical glucocorticoid treatment of psoriasis. Z Hautkr 1986;61: 161–166.

6   Editorial: The hazardous jungle of topical steroid. Lancet 1977;ii:487–488.

7   Weber E: Unerwünschte Wirkungen von Arzneimitteln: Ziele, Möglichkeiten und Schwächen der Erfassung. Münch Med Wochenschr 1989;131:97.

8   Hoigné R, Hottinger S: Monitoring adverse drug reactions in the post-marketing phase. Pharm Acta Helv 1988;1:2–12.

9   Rogers AS: Adverse drug events: Identification and attribution. Drug Intell Clin Pharm 1987;21: 915–920.

10 Urquhart J: Adverse drug reaction crisis management – before and after. Scrip 1388;19.

11 Avron J: Reporting drug side effects: Signals and noise. JAMA 1990;263:1823.

12 Scott HD, Thatcher-Renshaw A, Rosenbaum SE, Waters WJ Jr, Green M, Andrews LG, Faich GA: Physician reporting of adverse drug reactions. JAMA 1990;263:1785–1788.

13 Günther S: Systemische Nebenwirkungen durch Externkortikoide: Ergebnisse dermatologischer Untersuchungen an Kindern mit Neurodermitis. Z Hautkr 1976;51:838–844.

14 Akers WA: Risks of unoccluded topical steroids and clinical trials. Arch Dermatol 1980;116:786–788.

15 Hornstein OP, Wilsch L, Scheiber W: Hautschäden durch prolongierte externe Kortikosteroidanwendung: Eine statistische Häufigkeitsanalyse. Therapiewoche 1975;36:4905–4908.

16 Maurer P, Hoigné R, Hess T, Müller U, Wymann R, Jordi A, Maibach R: Systematische Erfassung der Nebenwirkungen von Arzneimitteln nach Markteinführung: Ergebnisse aus dem Komprehensiven Spital Drug Monitoring (CHDM) Bern. Münch Med Wochenschr 1989;131:105–108.

Th. Höhler, PhD, Clinical Research Department, Cassella-Riedel Pharma GmbH,
Hanauer Landstrasse 521, D–60386 Frankfurt (FRG)

Korting HC, Maibach HI (eds): Topical Glucocorticoids with Increased Benefit/Risk Ratio.
Curr Probl Dermatol. Basel, Karger, 1993, vol 21, pp 186–191

....

Topical Glucocorticoids and Anti-Infectives: A Rational Combination?

Helga Zienicke

Dermatologische Klinik und Poliklinik (Direktor: Prof. Dr. *G. Plewig*) der
Ludwig-Maximilians-Universität München, BRD

In 1952, Sulzberger and Witten [1] reported on the use of topical hydrocortisone for inflammatory skin disease, in particular atopic dermatitis. Later on, the question came up if the addition of an anti-infective might add to the efficacy of a topical drug in this indication. In fact, Leyden et al. [2] demonstrated that *Staphylococcus aureus* was often found in large quantities on lesional skin of atopics, the number of colony-forming units (CFU)/cm^2 exceeding 10^6 even if there were no clinical signs of superinfection. Moreover, clinical recovery if obtained was parallelled by a reduction of the microbial colonization. Hence, *S. aureus* seems to aggravate manifest atopic eczema.

Before this background, Marples et al. [3] investigated the use of the addition of neomycin plus gramicidin or nystatin to a triamcinolone-acetonide preparation in experimental skin infection. As expected by them they could demonstrate the superiority of the combination over the glucocorticoid alone. The data obtained by these experiments were strongly supported by corresponding findings in clinical trials as shown in table 1. Thus it seems to be quite clear that a glucocorticoid profits from the addition of an anti-infective. This has led to a very frequent use of such combinations in clinical practice as can be derived from topical data on prescription habits in Germany [8].

Recently, new topical glucocorticoids have been introduced into therapy, in particular those of the nonhalogenated double-ester type such as prednicarbate [9]. To assess the potential role of an anti-infective added to this drug, a double-blind multicenter trial in superinfected atopic eczema was performed.

Table 1. Efficacy of glucocorticoid antibiotic combinations versus glucocorticoid alone for eczema on clinical and microbiological grounds according to the literature

Group	Cases	Type of treatment (combination vs. corticosteroid alone)	Results	
			clinical outcome	pathogen elimination
Davis et al., 1968 [4]	27	betamethasone/ neomycin	identical	identical
Lloyd, 1969 [5]	45	fluocinolone acetonide/ neomycin	identical	combination better
Clark, 1974 [6]	40	fluocinolone acetonide/ neomycin	combination better	combination better
Leyden and Kligman, 1977 [7]	36	fluocinolone acetonide neomycin	combination better $p < 0.05$	combination better $p < 0.01$

Materials and Methods

This was a multicenter double-blind trial performed at six university or municipal departments of dermatology [for details, cf. 10]. The trial plan was approved by the local ethical committee of the major clinical investigator and conformed to the standards of the Declaration of Helsinki.

A total of 180 patients suffering from superinfected atopic eczema was to be enrolled. While atopic eczema was to be defined on clinical grounds by the doctor in charge, superinfection had to be proven by quantitative bacteriological analysis. More than 10^6 CFU of *S. aureus*/cm^2 were considered as minimum for final evaluation. If due to severity of superinfection systemic treatment was considered necessary, the patient was not to be included into the trial.

According to a random plan, each patient either received prednicarbate 0.25% cream representing an emulsion of the oil in water type (Dermatop® Creme, Cassella-Riedel Pharma, Frankfurt, FRG) or the identical drug differing just by the addition of the disinfectant didecyldimethylammoniumchloride at a concentration of 0.25% (Bardac 22®, Lonza, Grenzach, FRG). The preparations were supplied in blinded vessels.

One of the preparations was to be applied twice a day at all lesional sites except those of the face or the front part of the neck. Here only the vehicle preparation was to be used. After the initial treatment period of 5 days, either prednicarbate 0.25% cream or the corresponding vehicle was to be used according to the decision of the clinician in charge.

Visits of the patients were scheduled for days 0, 6, 20 and 34. The severity of the clinical signs redness, swelling, papulovesicles, vesicles, pustules, bullae, papules, status madidans, crusting and scaling were always to be judged using a score ranging from 1 (none) to 5 (very severe). In addition, adverse events had to be checked using a score from 1 (mild) to 3 (severe). Lack of success of initial treatment during the first 5 days led to the exclusion of the patient from further participation in the trial. After the initial treatment, general assess-

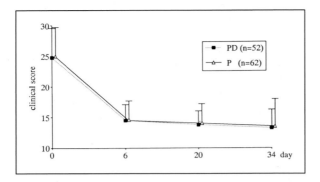

Fig. 1. Development of the total clinical score over time. PD = Prednicarbate plus didecyldimethylammoniumchloride; P = prednicarbate.

ment was also to be performed. Both the doctor and the patient had to judge efficacy, tolerability and cosmetic acceptability using a score ranging from 1 (excellent) to 4 (poor).

Bacterial colonization was checked at identical sites on days 0, 6 (or 7) and 34. For sampling, the detergent scrub method as described by Williamson and Kligman [11] was used. The washing fluids thus obtained were plated after systematic dilution on appropriate media and incubated. Plates carrying adequate numbers of suspicious looking colonies were used for counts. The identity of staphylococci was determined using standard methods including standardized tests for biochemical properties.

Both treatment groups were to be analyzed statistically with respect to data on demographics and success of treatment by Fisher's exact test. For the influence of treatment on the various skin lesions the Mantel-Haenszel test was chosen. Final evaluation was based on Fisher's test. $p < 0.05$ was considered to indicate a difference.

Results

A total of 54 male and 89 female patients could be recruited in 69 of whom the combination preparation was used. Eighteen patients had to be excluded from final evaluation as the *S. aureus* count gave a figure not exceeding $10^6/cm^2$. Eight patients were excluded as the age lay below 18 years. Eighteen patients could not be seen over the entire treatment period.

In general, there was a quick reduction of severity of disease particularly during the first 5 days. Yet there was no marked difference between the two treatment groups. The development of the total clinical score is depicted in figure 1. Figure 2a and b as well as figure 3a and b (color plate I) demonstrate the clinical picture before and after 5 days' treatment with prednicarbate plus didecyldi-

Table 2. Mean values and standard deviation (SD) of numbers of CFU/cm^2 of *S. aureus* in both treatment groups on days 0 and 6

Point of time	Group prednicarbate plus didecyl-dimethylammonium-chloride (n = 37)			Group prednicarbate (n = 44)		
	mean ± SD	min	max	mean ± SD	min	max
Initial visit (day 0)	50 ± 130	1	600	89 ± 200	1	890
First control visit (day 6)	34 ± 170	0.0006	1,000	7.1 ± 22	0	100

Table 3. Number of patients harboring *S. aureus* in both treatment groups on days 0, 6 and 34 in both treatment groups

Group	Point of time		
	initial visit (day 0)	first control visit (day 6)	last control visit (day 34)
Prednicarbate plus didecyldimethyl-ammoniumchloride	47	5	2
Prednicarbate	54	7	6 (p = 0.1)

methylammoniumchloride as well as prednicarbate cream alone. At the first follow-up, prednicarbate alone was considered efficacious by the physician in 87% of patients, the corresponding figure for the glucocorticoid anti-infective combination reading 92%. The corresponding figures for aesthetic acceptability and tolerability read 92/96 and 97/98%, respectively (p > 0.05).

In 1 patient after a few days itch and burning upon application of the medication was noted as well as vertigo which led to the discontinuation of application of the trial drug.

The number of CFU of *S. aureus* decreased rapidly in both treatment groups, in particular during the first 5 days. Mean values and standard deviation are given in table 2. Table 3 states the number of patients in whom *S. aureus* was found on days 0, 6 and 34 separately for both treatment groups.

Discussion

Even in most recent specialized textbooks on glucocorticoid treatment of skin disease, glucocorticoid antibiotic combinations are considered rational treatment for superinfected eczema [12]. At least with prednicarbate, however, the data of the present trial do not support the idea of an additional benefit of a glucocorticoid preparation for topical use if an anti-infective is added. This is in accordance with the results of a trial comparing betamethasone-valerate plus gentamicin to betamethasone-valerate alone [13]. Although in this case the pathogen was more efficaciously eliminated, the clinical outcome was not clearly better with the combination. It is worth considering that the clinical superiority of a glucocorticoid anti-infective combination was in particular demonstrated with triamcinolone-acetonide, as triamcinolone-acetonide is clearly less active as compared to both betamethasone-17-valerate and prednicarbate [14]. It is tempting to speculate that primarily weak topical glucocorticoids profit from the addition of the anti-infective while with medium potent topical glucocorticoids the anti-inflammatory potency is so great that this is the feature most relevant clinically. Reduction of inflammation might change the eco system of the skin surface to the worse for *S. aureus* quicker than the bacterium by itself can be markedly reduced due to direct antimicrobial activity of the dermatic.

Before this background the addition of an anti-infective to a medium potent topical glucocorticoid of the nonhalogenated double-ester type cannot be advocated currently. In this context it is of interest that the Bundesgesundheitsamt has recently discouraged the use of chlorquinaldol in a mixed preparation also including diflucortolone-21-valerate due to an inadequate benefit to risk ratio [15]. This particular glucocorticoid even has to be considered stronger than the congeners discussed so far.

In fact, there is also another interesting aspect of the present results: if the addition of an anti-infective does not definitely add to the clinical result of treatment of superinfected eczema as compared to the use of a medium potent glucocorticoid alone, superinfection should no longer be considered as a contraindication for such a compound. Due to the exclusion criteria in the present trial, no statement

Fig. 2. Microbial-laden atopic dermatitis at the lateral aspect of the neck of a 22-year-old female patient *a* before treatment with the number of CFU of *S. aureus*/cm² amounting to 3.8×10^6, and *b* after 5 days of treatment with the prednicarbate anti-infective combination, the number of CFU of *S. aureus*/cm² amounting to 14.7×10^6.

Fig. 3. Microbial-laden atopic dermatitis at the left thigh of a 19-year-old female patient *a* before and *b* after 5 days' treatment with prednicarbate cream, the number of CFU of *S. aureus*/cm² amounting to 46×10^6 and 0, respectively.

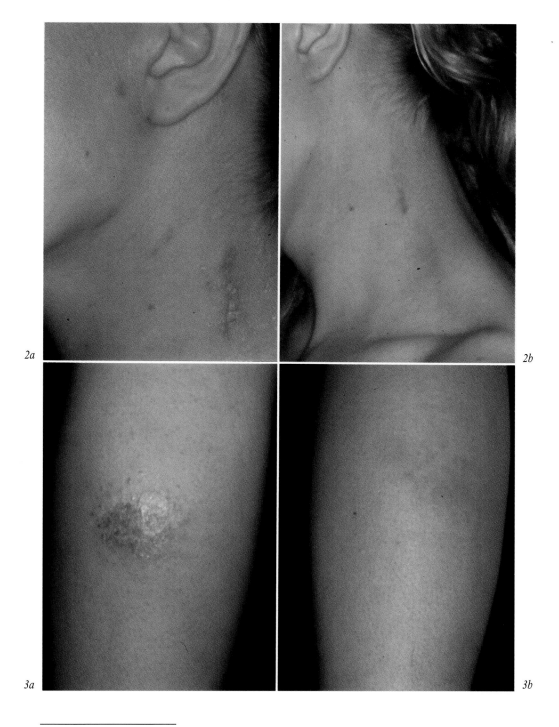

2a 2b

3a 3b

Topical Glucocorticoids and Anti-Infectives   Plate I

can be made as to cases of severe superinfection considered to require systemic antibiotic treatment. If such a treatment, however, is not mandatory, the doctor in charge of a given patient can rely on drugs like prednicarbate alone.

The course of disease upon the application of the trial medication during the 5 days always including prednicarbate 0.25% corresponds to previous findings as to the clinical efficacy in eczema [16].

References

1   Sulzberger MB, Witten VH: Effect of topically applied compound F in selected dermatoses. J Invest Dermatol 1952;19:101–102.
2   Leyden JJ, Marples RR, Kligman A: *Staphylococcus aureus* in the lesions of atopic dermatitis. Br J Dermatol 1974;90:525–530.
3   Marples RR, Rebora A, Kligman AM: Topical steroid-antibiotic combinations. Assay of use in experimentally induced human infections. Arch Dermatol 1973;108:237–240.
4   Davis CM, Fulghum DD, Taplin D: The value of neomycin in a neomycin-steroid cream. J Am Med Assoc 1968;203:136–138.
5   Lloyd KM: The value of neomycin in topical corticosteroid preparations. South Med J 1969;62: 94–96.
6   Clark RF: The case for corticosteroid-antibiotic combinations. Cutis 1974;14:737–741.
7   Leyden JJ, Kligman AM: The case for steroid-antibiotic combinations. Br J Dermatol 1977;96: 179–187.
8   Fricke U: Dermatika; in Schwabe U, Paffrath D (eds): Arzneiverordnungsreport '92. Stuttgart, Fischer, 1992, pp 169–194.
9   Drebinger K, Hoehler T: Prednicarbate; in Maibach HI, Surber C (eds): Topical Corticosteroids. Basel, Karger, 1992, pp 480–493.
10 Korting HC, Zienicke H, Braun-Falco O, Bork K, Milbradt R, Nolting S, Schöpf E, Tronnier H: Modern topical glucocorticoids and anti-infectives for super-infected atopic eczema: Do prednicarbate and didecyldimethylammoniumchloride form a rational combination? In preparation.
11 Williamson P, Kligman AM: A new method for the quantitative investigation of cutaneous bacteria. J Invest Dermatol 1965;45:498–503.
12 Clement M, du Vivier A: Praxis der kutanen Steroidtherapie. Berlin, Blackwell Überreuter, 1990.
13 Wachs GN, Maibach HI: Co-operative double-blind trial of an antibiotic corticoid combination in impetiginized atopic dermatitis. Br J Dermatol 1976;95:323–328.
14 Niedner R: Richtlinien zur Anwendung externer Glukokortikoide. Med Welt 1989;40:703–705.
15 Arzneimittelinformationsstelle der ABDA: Chlorquinaldol (Stoffcharakteristik): Pharm Zeitung 1991;136:1741.
16 Vogt HJ, Hoehler T: Controlled studies of intraindividual and interindividual design for comparing corticosteroids clinically; in Christophers E, Schöpf E, Kligman AM, Stoughton RB (eds): Topical Corticosteroid Therapy. A Novel Approach to Safer Drugs. New York, Raven Press, 1988, pp 169–179.

Helga Zienicke, MD, Dermatologische Klinik und Poliklinik der
Ludwig-Maximilians-Universität, Frauenlobstrasse 9–11, D–80337 München (FRG)

Korting HC, Maibach HI (eds): Topical Glucocorticoids with Increased Benefit/Risk Ratio.
Curr Probl Dermatol. Basel, Karger, 1993, vol 21, pp 192–201

....

Topical Glucocorticoids: What Has Been Achieved? What Is Still to Be Done?

M. Schäfer-Korting

Pharmakologisches Institut für Naturwissenschaftler der
Johann-Wolfgang-Goethe-Universität, Frankfurt/Main, BRD

In the last decade, not only scientists and physicians but also the patients became more and more aware of adverse drug reactions. Thus, with many kinds of drug treatment an improvement of the benefit/risk ratio is looked for [1, 2]. The very unfavourable outcome of the Cardiac Arrhythmia Suppression Trial (CAST) requiring even an abrupt stop of two treatment arms induced a serious reconsideration of anti-arrhythmic therapy [3]. Above that, the benefit/risk ratio for the topical and systemic use of β_2-adrenoceptor agonists has been discussed recently [4], and animal experiments were performed to improve the therapeutic index of diuretics [5].

Adverse Drug Reactions

Despite unquestionable efficacy, today the use of topical glucocorticoids is limited by the fear of side-effects [6, 7]. These include numerous local and systemic reactions varying from mild to life-threatening. Besides skin atrophy a suppression of the hypothalamic-pituitary-adrenal axis is mostly feared. Diminution of skin thickness due to the inhibition of keratinocyte and fibroblast proliferation occurs rapidly in almost every patient receiving potent topical steroids. After a certain point, the dermis can be irreversibly damaged which becomes obvious by striae formation. Suppression of the hypothalamic-pituitary-adrenal axis is a rare but severe event; deaths have occurred. Much effort is taken to reduce these events.

In theory, an improved benefit/risk ratio can be obtained by chemical modifications of the drug molecule as well as by the optimisation of vehicles and therapeutic regimens. Whereas only recently some effort was taken to develop improved vehicles, optimisation of the drug molecule and the therapeutic regimens is tried since the beginning of the topical steroid era. Indeed, several principles – recently summarised by Niedner [8] – have been established which proved very valuable.

Optimisation of Therapeutic Regimens

To avoid unnecessary adverse drug reactions it is of utmost importance to use these agents only in steroid-sensitive dermatoses and to use a steroid of the weakest potency which will clear the disease. Above that, it is well known that the horny layer does not only act as a penetration barrier for glucocorticoids but also has a depot function [9, 10]. This allows the reduction of the application frequency of these agents. Base preparations applied inbetween two steroid applications favour drug penetration to the viable skin and thus enhance activity. There is, however, still a considerable lack of information which treatment schedule – e.g. glucocorticoids once daily, 5 times a week or even once a week – fits best to which steroid. Pertinent research should be continued.

To adapt the regimen to the severity of the dermatosis also the induction of treatment with a potent steroid and the switch to a less potent one after the acute phase has been advocated. This concept is, however, not unquestionable, since there is a major damage of the horny layer during the acute phase which favours steroid penetration and thus adverse drug reactions. During the healing process the penetration barrier re-establishes. Therefore, steroids with reduced strength then may not be adequate.

Since the pharmacokinetic studies performed by Feldmann and Maibach [11], the extensive variations of glucocorticoid absorption depending on the thickness of the horny layer are well known. Therefore, mild steroids and cream preparations are favoured for dermatoses of the face and intertriginous areas.

It also turned out very rapidly that there are special risk groups for adverse drug reactions. These are infants due to their thinner horny layer and patients with liver disease because of an impaired glucocorticoid metabolism. Treating these with mild to moderate steroids thus reduces the risk of side-effects.

Molecular Modifications

Besides the optimisation of the treatment schedule, there has been an intensive search for drugs with an improved therapeutic index, and this is still going on. Aims in the development were to reduce skin atrophy and/or adrenal suppression as compared to equipotent conventional steroids. Thus, a steroid highly effective against inflammation with a low risk of skin thinning in particular is desired especially for atopic eczema. With respect to psoriasis vulgaris an improvement of the benefit/risk ratio is even more difficult to obtain, since antipsoriatic activity and skin atrophy seem to be linked to the antimitotic effect.

Despite large variations in potency, an improvement of the therapeutic index by chemical derivatisation of the steroid structure most often failed. Wanted and unwanted effects in general run in parallel. Potency is increased, e.g., by the formation of 17-esters or 16,17-acetonides due to an increased receptor binding and improved tissue penetration. The latter holds true also with respect to 21-esters. 17,21-Diesters have a reduced receptor binding as compared to the 17-monoesters [12] but are rapidly hydrolysed in the skin [13] and thus act as a prodrug.

Today there is no indication for differences in the physicochemical properties of glucocorticoid receptors [6] excluding improved selectivity by enhanced affinity for special receptor subtypes. This opinion, however, may be revised in the future, if additional nuclear receptors will be discovered as it has been the case with retinoic acid [14, 15] – glucocorticoid and retinoic acid receptors belonging to the same receptor family.

There are, however, some agents which seem to have an improved benefit/risk ratio [16] and interesting results have been presented. Yet today pharmacokinetic instead of pharmacodynamic reasons are considered relevant in this respect. In theory, reduced local and systemic side effects are obtained by drug moieties sensitive to metabolism in the deeper skin layers to inactive or less active metabolites. This has to occur after the induction of the desired effect by the native substance in the upper strata of viable skin. Systemic adverse reactions are also reduced by a rapid metabolism in blood or liver which have a much higher enzyme activity as compared to the skin [17].

Today we have several non-halogenated glucocorticoid double esters and we have one derivative of the 21-carboxylic acid esters, fluocortin butyl, on the market. Other 21-carboxyl methyl esters [18] and 16-carboxy esters and amides of prednisolone are under investigation as are mometasone and thiosteroids [19, 20].

Fluocortin butyl is the first glucocorticoid strictly adhering to the concept of drug targeting [21]. It is derived from the steroid C-21 acid by esterification with butanol [22] leading to an inverse arrangement of the acid and alcohol components within the side chain. Whereas corticosteroid esters with inverse arrangements are moderately active, the C-21 acid has no affinity for the glucocorticoid receptor and shows no activity in vivo. Thus, fluocortin butyl is inactivated after absorption into the skin by esterases excluding systemic effects but largely at the expense of potency.

On the market there are also some non-halogenated double esters of hydrocortisone and prednisolone. Among these, prednicarbate has been introduced first and evaluated most carefully. Recent investigations proved not prednicar-

Table 1. Receptor affinities of prednicarbate and its metabolites as well as betamethasone and its valerate esters

	Prednicarbate[a] [23]	Betamethasone[b] [12]
17,21-Double ester	0.04	4.8
17-Monoester	74	13
21-Monoester	–	1.4
Non-ester moiety	14	2.2

[a] Dexamethasone = 100.
[b] Hydrocortisone = 1.

bate itself but prednisolone 17-ethyl carbonate to have the highest glucocorticoid receptor affinity (table 1) [23]. The results of phase I studies and the influence on skin thickness have been reported. Non-occlusive application of prednicarbate 0.25% cream induces only a minor reduction of skin thickness as compared to betamethasone 17-valerate [24, 25]. Since, however, occlusion leads to major skin thinning [24, 26] as well as adrenal suppression [26], the increase in the therapeutic index is not an absolute but only a relative one. Fast absorption overcomes the inactivation process. Therefore, measurements of skin atrophy should be performed for each vehicle. Other non-halogenated double esters reported to have an improved therapeutic index are hydrocortisone aceponate and hydrocortisone 17-butyrate 21-propionate [16, 27].

In addition to the glucocorticoid receptor affinities of prednisolone derivatives, table 1 gives also the receptor affinities of betamethasone and its valerate esters. Also betamethasone 17-valerate affinity declines sharply, if the 17-valerate ester is hydrolysed [12]. The higher atrophogenic potential of betamethasone 17-valerate as compared to prednicarbate suggests a lower hydrolysis rate in the skin.

Rapid hydrolysis in the skin does not apply to 6-methylprednisolone aceponate either. This is another non-halogenated prednisolone derivative coming to the market in the near future. Detailed metabolic studies by Täuber and Rost [28] showed a rapid activation to the 17-propionate in the skin which is hydrolysed only slowly in this tissue. As with prednicarbate, the 17-monoester has a much higher glucocorticoid receptor affinity as compared to the 17,21-double ester [28].

Another recent result of the efforts to separate wanted and unwanted effects of topically applied glucocorticoids has been the development of mometasone furoate, a chlorinated congener. In patients treated for psoriasis vulgaris mometasone furoate has not induced more overt skin atrophy than hydrocortisone 1%

ointment despite better efficacy [29]. To obtain objective data of skin thickness and to detect subtle signs of cutaneous atrophy, investigations with more sensitive techniques are necessary. Yet the results obtained suggest that the development of topical glucocorticoids with an improved benefit/risk ratio may be possible even facing psoriasis vulgaris and with a halogenated glucocorticoid.

A further approach is represented by the recently developed drug tipredane and other labile alkylthio-groups on C-17. The evaluation of these steroids is based on the observation of a high affinity of various sulphur-containing drugs to the skin and rapid oxidation to sulphoxides and sulphones. Thus, systemic availability is low, whereas local anti-inflammatory effects resemble those of other moderately potent to potent glucocorticoids [19, 30]. Within the thiosteroids CSK-802 seems to be most interesting due to its unique active transport by the fMLP receptor into inflammatory cells. This receptor protein is not expressed by the other cells. The results thus suggest that an improved benefit/risk ratio may be obtainable with CSK-802 [T. Höhler, pers. communication]. Moreover, it stimulates the search for other steroids with an improved therapeutic index.

Benefit/Risk Ratio of Topical Glucocorticoids

Since there are by now several congeners reported to induce less adverse drug reactions as compared to equipotent conventional glucocorticoids [16], we urgently need a technique to quantify the benefit/risk ratio. Presently there is no sound basis for a ranking. To make a proposal, I suggest to compare the ratios of drug activity and atrophogenicity, the most relevant adverse drug reaction. Both can be determined in healthy volunteers, thus avoiding laborious trials in patients which are also hampered by large scatter of data. The atrophogenic potential is evaluated by ultrasound measurement of skin thickness following steroid application for up to 6 weeks [25, 27]. Potency is derived from one of the standard methods for human pharmacology of topical steroids, e.g. the vasoconstrictor assay, ultraviolet UV erythema test, Wells test or tuberculin test [31, 32].

The ratios for betamethasone 17-valerate, hydrocortisone aceponate and prednicarbate can be calculated from data already presented [27, 33]. Skin thickness was determined in two separate experiments following the cream and ointment preparations; results are rather close (table 2). Drug activity was determined by the vasoconstrictor assay with and without occlusion as well as the UV erythema test. Ratios are based on the sums of visual scores and percent reduction of skin thickness. The results (table 2) show a clearly higher ratio for the glucocorticoids of the non-halogenated double-ester type (hydrocortisone aceponate and prednicarbate) as compared to the betamethasone 17-valerate. More studies, however, are needed to substantiate these differences by confirmatory statistics.

Schäfer-Korting

Table 2. Benefit/risk ratio of prednicarbate (PC), hydrocortisone aceponate (HC-AP) and betamethasone 17-valerate (BMV) derived from the activity in the vasoconstrictor assay (VC) and UV erythema test [33] and the reduction of skin thickness in healthy volunteers [27]

	PC	HC-AP	BMV
Activity: sum score			
VC (occluded)	16	21	14
VC (non-occluded)	6	25	15
UV erythema test	8	25	10
Percent reduction of skin thickness			
Ointment/cream	11.2/8.2	10.6/–	17.2/14.7
Benefit/risk ratio			
VC (occluded)	1.4/2.0	2.0	0.81/1.0
VC (non-occluded)	0.54/0.73	2.4	0.87/1.0
UV erythema test	0.71/1.0	0.94	0.58/0.68

– = Not done.

Vehicle Effects

To make topical steroid treatment more tolerable in the future, also a closer look at the vehicles seems advisable. Investigations with indometacin by Loth demonstrated a major alteration in drug distribution between viable epidermis and dermis by the addition of various penetration enhancers to a standard triglyceride ointment base (Softisan 378). The incorporation of 10% medium-chain triglycerides (Myglyol® 812) or oleyl oleate (Cetiol®) increase the indometacin level in the viable epidermis by 49 and 21% without a parallel increase of the dermal concentration. There are other penetration enhancers, as for example octanol, favouring indometacin penetration to the dermis [34]. Thus, it seems possible to increase glucocorticoid concentrations at the site of wanted effects without a parallel increase at sites where it is not needed.

Liposomes

Besides penetration enhancers also liposome encapsulation may be a valuable tool. Recently we compared a liposomal preparation of betamethasone 17,21-dipropionate 0.039% to a 0.064% commercial propylene glycol gel in a

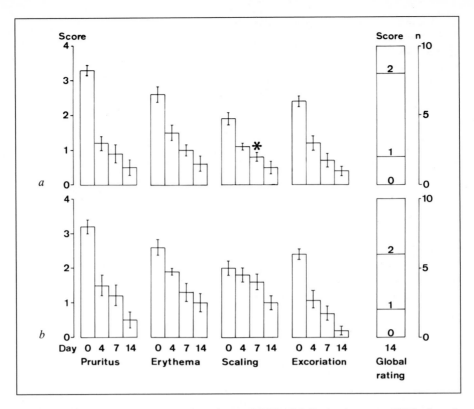

Fig. 1. Betamethasone 17,21-dipropionate (BDP) trial. Rating (mean ± SEM) of pruritus, erythema, scaling and excoriation in 10 patients with atopic eczema before the study (day 0) and on three follow-up visits, as well as global treatment response on the last treatment day. *a* Liposome-encapsulated BDP. * p ≤0.05. *b* BDP reference gel. [From ref. 39 with permission.]

double-blind, randomised paired trial lasting 14 days in 10 patients with atopic eczema and 10 patients with psoriasis vulgaris [35]. In eczema, liposome encapsulation increased betamethasone 17,21-dipropionate efficacy (fig. 1), whereas no improvement was seen in psoriasis vulgaris. Due to the supposed linkage of antipsoriatic activity and skin atrophy to the antiproliferative effect, liposome encapsulation may improve the benefit/risk ratio of topically applied glucocorticoids with respect to eczema. Moreover, pharmacokinetic studies with liposome-encapsulated triamcinolone acetonide [36, 37] and hydrocortisone [38] indicate higher drug levels in the skin and a lower systemic availability which should mean less systemic side-effects.

In this context, it is also of interest that liposomes are made of phospholipids acting as penetration enhancers, even if not formulated as liposomes. In the near future, even epidermal lipids are feasible as glucocorticoid vehicles and may further reduce adverse reactions. In fact, it is most interesting to see that the reduction of skin thickness by prednicarbate and hydrocortisone aceponate is also seen with the respective vehicles [25, 27].

Dose-Response Relationship

To my mind also dose-response curves of anti-inflammatory and atrophogenic effects of conventional steroids should be studied in detail. At present, the concentrations are based only on the wanted actions and are usually on the plateau of the dose-response curve. Our most recent data suggest that this also holds true for prednicarbate cream [33]. While this overdosage is of no major concern with respect to the well-tolerated prednicarbate cream, a dosage reduction may be most useful with respect to conventional steroids, as for example betamethasone 17-valerate, clobetasol 17-propionate or desoximetasone. Moreover, it is not excluded that patients with an impaired penetration barrier will take a profit also from a reduced prednicarbate concentration.

Combined Treatment with Glucocorticoids and Retinoids

Finally, another approach to increase the benefit/risk ratio of topical glucocorticoids by minimising the atrophogenic potential could be the simultaneous application of retinoic acid, which has the ability of inducing epidermal hyperplasia, enhancing collagen synthesis, even in steroid-inhibited wound healing. Experiments in animals have shown a prevention of glucocorticoid-induced skin atrophy by pretreatment with all-*trans*-retinoic acid without a decrease in the anti-inflammatory effect [39]. Preliminary results in humans also look stimulating [40]. Besides tretinoin, also the topical application of 12% ammonium lactate solution may mitigate cutaneous atrophy [41].

Conclusion

Clinical and experimental data available so far suggest an improved benefit/risk ratio of some topical glucocorticoids with respect to the most important side effects skin atrophy and adrenal suppression. Yet there seems to be the potential for further improvements in the future. To my mind there is, however, currently no chance to reduce the other local side effects as for example steroid-induced rosacea which seems to be linked to the constriction of blood vessels in the upper strata of the corium.

References

1 Palminteri R: Benefit/risk ratio of new drugs: For whom? J R Soc Med 1988;81:155–157.
2 Wolverton SE: Monitoring for adverse effects from systemic drugs used in dermatology. J Am Acad Dermatol 1992;26:661–679.
3 Anderson JL: Reassessment of benefit-risk ratio and treatment algorithms for antiarrhythmic drug therapy after the Cardiac Arrythmia Suppression Trial. J Clin Pharmacol 1990;30:981–989.
4 Ziment I: Risk/benefit ratio of long-term treatment with β_2-adrenoceptor agonists. Lung 1990(suppl):168–176.
5 Zhi J, Levy G: Optimization of the therapeutic index by adjustment of the rate of drug administration or use of drug combinations: Exploratory studies of diuretics. Pharmacol Res 1990;7:697–702.
6 Bateman DN: Clinical pharmacology of topical steroids: in Greaves MW, Shuster S (eds): Pharmacology of the Skin II. Berlin, Springer, 1989, pp 239–249.
7 Robertson DB, Maibach HI: Topical glucocorticoids; in Schleimer RP, Claman HN, Oronsky A (eds): Anti-Inflammatory Steroid Action. Basic and Clinical Aspects. San Diego, Academic Press, 1989, pp 494–524.
8 Niedner R: Grundlagen einer rationalen Therapie mit externen Glukokortikosteroiden. Hautarzt 1991;42:337–346.
9 Vickers CFH: Existence of reservoir in the stratum corneum: Experimental proof. Arch Dermatol 1963;88:72–75.
10 Stoughton RB: Dimethylsulfoxide (DMSO) induction of a steroid reservoir in human skin. Arch Dermatol 1965;91:657–660.
11 Feldmann RJ, Maibach HI:Regional variation in percutaneous penetration of ^{14}C-cortisol in man. J Invest Dermatol 1967;48:181.
12 Ponec M, Kempenaar J, Shroot B, Caron JC: Glucocorticoids: Binding affinity and lipophilicity. J Pharm Sci 1986;75:973–975.
13 Cheung YW, LiWanPo A, Irwin WJ: Cutaneous biotransformation as a parameter in the modulation of the activity of topical corticosteroids. Int J Pharm 1985;26:175–189.
14 Petkovich M, Brand NJ, Krust A, Chambon P: A human retinoic acid receptor which belongs to the family of nuclear receptors. Nature 1987;330:444–450.
15 Mangelsdorf DJ, Ong ES, Dyck JA, Evans RM: Nuclear receptor that identifies a novel retinoic acid response pathway. Nature 1990;345:224–229.
16 Korting HC, Kerscher MJ, Schäfer-Korting M: Topical glucocorticoids with improved benefit-risk ratio – Do they exist? J Am Acad Dermatol 1992;27:87–92.
17 Täuber U: Drug metabolism in the skin: Advantages and disadvantages; in Hadgraft N, Guy RH (eds): Transdermal Drug Delivery. Developmental Issues and Research Initiatives. New York, Dekker, 1989, pp 99–112.
18 DiPetrillo T, Lee H, Cutroneo KR: Anti-inflammatory adrenal steroids that neither inhibit skin collagen synthesis nor cause dermal atrophy. Arch Dermatol 1984;120:878–883.
19 Milioni K: Topical anti-inflammatory thiosteroids; in Maibach HI, Surber C (eds): Topical Corticosteroids. Basel, Karger, 1992, pp 142–153.
20 Taraporewala IB, Kim HP, Heiman AS, Lee HJ: A novel class of local anti-inflammatory steroids. Arzneimittel-Forschung 1989;39:21–25.
21 Laurent H, Gerhards E, Wiechert R: Synthese von 6α-Fluor-11β-hydroxy-16α-methyl-3,20-dioxo-1,4-pregnadien-21-säure-butylester (Fluocortin-butylester). Arzneimittel-Forschung 1977;27:2187–2188.

22 Herz-Hübner U, Täuber U: Metabolisierung von Flucortin-butylester in der Haut von Meerschweinchen und Mensch. Arzneimittel-Forschung 1977;27:2226–2229.

23 Pörtner M, Möllmann H, Rohdewald P: Glucocorticoid receptors in human synovial tissue and relative receptor affinities of glucocorticoid-21-esters. Pharm Res 1988;5:623–627.

24 Dykes PJ, Hill S, Marks R: Assessment of the atrophogenicity potential of corticosteroids by ultrasound and by epidermal biopsy under occlusive and nonocclusive conditions; in Christophers E, Schöpf E, Kligman AM, Stoughton RB (eds): Topical Corticosteroid Therapy. A Novel Approach to Safer Drugs. New York, Raven Press, 1988, pp 111–118.

25 Korting HC, Vieluf D, Kerscher M: 0.25% Prednicarbate cream and the corresponding vehicle induce less skin atrophy than 0.1% betamethasone-17-valerate cream and 0.05% clobetasol-17-propionate cream. Eur J Clin Pharmacol 1992;42:159–161.

26 Maas-Irslinger R, Breitbart EW: Vergleichende Untersuchung der systemischen und lokalen Nebenwirkungen von Prednicarbat und herkömmlichen halogenierten Kortikosteroiden; in Macher E, Knop J, Bröcker EB (eds): Jahrbuch der Dermatologie 1988. Münster, Biermann, 1989, pp 123–129.

27 Korting HC: Topical glucocorticoids and thinning of normal skin as to be assessed by ultrasound; in Korting HC, Maibach HI (eds): Topical Glucocorticoids with Increased Benefit/Risk Ratio. Curr Probl Dermatol. Basel, Karger, 1993, pp 114–121.

28 Täuber U, Rost KL: Esterase activity of the skin including species variations; in Shroot B, Schaefer H (eds): Skin Pharmacokinetics. Pharmacol Skin. Basel, Karger, 1987, vol. 1, pp 170–183.

29 Katz HI, Prawer SE, Watson MJ, Scull TA, Peets EA: Mometasone furoate ointment 0.1% vs. hydrocortisone ointment 1.0% in psoriasis. Int J Dermatol 1989;28:342–344.

30 Devlin RG, Dean A, Kripalani KJ, Taylor JR, Sugermann AA: Percutaneous absorption and adrenal suppressive potency of tipredane, a new topical corticosteroid. J Toxicol, Cutan Ocul Toxicol 1986;5:35–43.

31 Wendt H, Frosch PJ: Clinico-Pharmacological Models for the Assay of Topical Corticoids. Basel, Karger, 1982.

32 Schalla W, Schorning S: Potency assessment of topical corticoids in the vasoconstrictor assay and on tuberculin induced inflammation. Skin Pharmacol 1991;4:191–204.

33 Kerscher M: Suppression of induced inflammation in man; in Korting HC, Maibach HI (eds): Topical Glucocorticoids with Increased Benefit/Risk Ratio. Curr Probl Dermatol. Basel, Karger, 1993, vol 21, pp 97–106.

34 Loth H: Skin permeability. Methods Find Exp Clin Pharmacol 1989;11:155–164.

35 Korting HC, Zienicke H, Schäfer-Korting M, Braun-Falco O: Liposome encapsulation improves efficacy of betamethasone dipropionate in atopic eczema but not in psoriasis vulgaris. Eur J Clin Pharmacol 1990;39:349–351.

36 Mezei M, Gulasekharam V: Liposomes – A selective drug delivery system for the topical route of administration. I. Lotion dosage form. Life Sci 1980;26:1473–1477.

37 Mezei M, Gulasekharam V: Liposomes – A selective drug delivery system for the topical route of administration: Gel dosage form. J Pharm Pharmacol 1982;34:473–474.

38 Wohlrab W, Lasch J, Taube KM, Wozniak KD: Hautpermeation von liposomal inkorporiertem Hydrocortison. Pharmazie 1989;44:333–335.

39 Lesnik RH, Mezick JA, Capetola R, Kligman LH: Topical all-trans-retinoic acid prevents corticosteroid-induced skin atrophy without abrogating the anti-inflammatory effect. J Am Acad Dermatol 1989;21:186–190.

40 Kligman LH, Schwartz E, Lesnik RH, Mezick JA: Topical tretinoin prevents corticosteroid-induced atrophy without lessening the anti-inflammatory effect; in Korting HC, Maibach HI (eds): Topical Glucocorticoids with Increased Benefit/Risk Ratio. Curr Probl Dermatol. Basel, Karger, 1993, vol 21, pp 79–88.

41 Lavker RM, Kaidbey K, Leyden JJ: Effects of topical ammonium lactate on cutaneous atrophy from a potent topical corticosteroid. J Am Acad Dermatol 1992;26:535–544.

PD Dr. M. Schäfer-Korting, Pharmakologisches Institut für Naturwissenschaftler
der Johann-Wolfgang-Goethe-Universität, Theodor-Stern-Kai 7, D–60596 Frankfurt/M (FRG)

Subject Index

disease responsiveness 157–159
effects
   fibroblasts 73–78, 122
   Langerhans cells 68–71
   sudden withdrawal 125
halogenation, effects on lipophilicity
   3, 5, 9
mechanism of action 6, 7, 20, 21, 122
partitioning, skin 57, 58
patch testing 171, 172
percutaneous absorption, *see* Absorption, percutaneous
potency
   effects
      administration route 147–155
      anti-infectives 186–191
      binding affinity 26, 27
      cellular uptake 26, 27
      dilution 159, 160
      liposome encapsulation 197–199
      metabolism, compounds 57, 160,
         194
      occlusion 48, 51, 132, 137
      penetration enhancers 92–94
      skin permeability 6, 27
      steroid
         clearance 27
         structure 3–5, 23–25, 137,
            193–196
      measurements 89, 90
receptors, *see* Receptors, glucocorticoid
side effects, therapy
   adverse drug reactions 180–184, 182,
      193
   allergic contact dermatitis 125
   infection masking 123, 125
   peripheral 7, 8, 11, 18, 79, 97, 114,
      115, 123–125, 192
   retinoid reversal 79–86, 199
   systemic 8, 11, 122, 123, 192
Glycosaminoglycans, effects
   retinoids 84, 85
   steroids 84, 85, 79

Halcinonide
   brand names 163, 164
   development 2

potency 5
sensitizing potential 176–178
Hydrocortisone
   anti-inflammatory activity 98, 100, 101,
      104, 105
   brand names 161
   conformation 13, 17
   history, clinical use 1
   liposome encapsulation effect, efficacy
      198
   metabolic deactivation 12, 13
   penetration, modified skin 51–54
   potency 5
   skin thinning 126–131, 137
   structure 3, 4, 13
   urea effects, penetration 166

Langerhans cells
   functions 68
   glucocorticoid effects
      cell
         function 70, 71
         number 70
      HLA class II molecule expression
         68–70
   percentage of total epidermal cells 68
   stimulation, psoriasis 68
   ultraviolet B light effects 70
Liposomes, encapsulation effect on drug
   efficacy 197–199
Living skin equivalent
   defined 61
   metabolism, corticosteroids 61–66
Loteprednol etabonate
   conformation 13, 17
   half-life 18
   potency 16–18
   side effects 18

Mometasone furoate, development 2

Nandrolone, absorption, psoriasis 52
Neomycin, eczema therapy, steroids 186,
   187
Nonsteroidal anti-inflammatory drugs, *see*
   Bufexamac